LOSS IN PREGNANCY

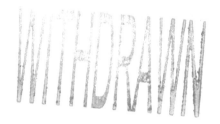

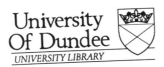

LOSS IN PREGNANCY
Guidelines for Midwives

Marie McDonald
RGN, RM, ADM

Head of Midwifery and Gynaecology Nursing
Clinical Services Manager
Women's Health Service
Lewisham Hospitals NHS Trust
London
UK

Baillière Tindall
London Philadelphia Toronto Sydney Tokyo

Baillière Tindall 24–28 Oval Road
London NW1 7DX

The Curtis Center
Independence Square West
Philadelphia, PA 19106-3399, USA

Harcourt Brace & Company
55 Horner Avenue
Toronto, Ontario, M8Z 4X6, Canada

Harcourt Brace & Company, Australia
30–52 Smidmore Street
Marrickville
NSW 2204, Australia

Harcourt Brace & Company, Japan
Ichibancho Central Building
Chiyoda-ku, Tokyo 102, Japan

This book is printed on acid-free paper

A catalogue record for this book is available from the British Library

ISBN 0-7020-1742-6

Typeset by Paston Press Ltd, Loddon, Norfolk
Printed and bound in Great Britain by WBC Book Manufacturers Ltd, Bridgend,
Mid Glamorgan

CONTENTS

Introduction

The antenatal care of women during pregnancy is designed to detect conditions of relevance to both mother and her fetus.

(Terry 1990)

Antenatal care has been an accepted philosophy for women in the United Kingdom since the turn of the century. The basic pattern was established in 1929 by the Minister for Health and the design has continued, virtually unchallenged, for over fifty years. The traditional pattern of attendance consists of monthly visits to a midwife or doctor until 28 weeks gestation, increasing to fortnightly until 36 weeks and then weekly until the baby is born. In their report *Changing Childbirth* the Expert Maternity Group said that:

The system of antenatal care currently in place is cumbersome and a source of concern to professionals and pregnant women alike. The Expert Group strongly recommends that a survey of existing practice is undertaken by purchasers, providers and professionals on a regular basis.

(Department of Health 1993)

Maternal health is assessed by urinalysis, measuring blood pressure and through a range of serum screening tests. Fetal well-being is determined by palpation of the abdomen to assess growth, position and number of babies, by ultrasound scanning to confirm findings and by auscultation of the heartbeat (Tew 1995; Department of Health 1993). Labour generally commences between 38 and 42 weeks gestation and the woman gives birth to a healthy baby or babies. The purpose of providing antenatal care is to detect any deviations from this normal progress, which can occur at any time during the pregnancy; deviations could range from minor disorders such as urinary tract infection, to serious complications such as pre-eclampsia. The aim, for medical and midwifery staff, is to correct the problem in order for pregnancy to proceed normally.

Multiple pregnancies are diagnosed when there is more than one fetus *in utero*. It is generally accepted that the greater the number of fetuses the higher will be their morbidity and mortality. Multiple pregnancies have a mortality rate three to four times that of a singleton pregnancy (Beischer 1988). The pregnancy may be the result of a fertility programme and follow a long history of infertility. Alternatively, it may be spontaneous and present problems of increasing the family in multiples. Regardless of the setting and history, the inevitable response by society to multiple pregnancies is that they are special (MacDonald 1994).

Unfortunately, the conclusion to the pregnancy is not always the expected outcome. A number of factors may result in complications throughout the antenatal period and in the possible death of the baby. Alternatively, the deliberate termination of a pregnancy may follow the detection of a fetal abnormality or a life-threatening maternal condition.

To the parents and family the terminology surrounding perinatal loss can be upsetting. Words and phrases such as 'abortion' and retained products of conception and fetus can cause distress and increased confusion over what is happening to them. Caring for parents in this situation presents many challenges for the staff, both in psychological terms and for the practical management around the birth and beyond. Apparently minor details such as gestational age have a much wider significance in law than many realise.

On 1 October 1992 the Stillbirth (Definition) Act reduced the age of viability from 28 to 24 weeks, a limit originally defined in the 1929 Infant Life (Preservation) Act (Stillbirth (Definition) Act 1992). Babies born before the age of legal viability are classified as pre-viable, have no legal status and are termed miscarriages. A stillbirth certificate is issued for babies born dead after 24 weeks (Dimond 1993). When signs of life are present in the pre-viable baby, he or she is registered as a live birth and certified as a neonatal death.

One of the purposes of this book is to consider the various types of perinatal loss that can occur during pregnancy, the management of the death and the practical details which are necessary for each. In all events there will be an inevitable overlap, for example in the taking of photographs, therefore these areas will be considered as a whole.

EXPERIENCING ANTENATAL LOSS

Spontaneous abortion, therapeutic termination of pregnancy and stillbirths can all be caused by a variety of factors. Threats to the pregnancy can present in a number of ways. How does the women know when she is at risk? How is the decision made to refer certain women to prenatal diagnosis? What happens when the diagnosis of death is confirmed? Each situation and every individual presents its own set of problems and questions. For some situations there are clear answers, for others it will depend on a number of factors. In dealing with problems that arise it is important that the woman and her partner have confidence in the nurses, midwives and doctors who are caring for her. Advice from other, experienced colleagues should always be sought and given as appropriate.

REFERENCES

Beischer NA (1988) Multiple pregnancy. In (NA Beischer & EV Mackay, eds.) *Obstetrics and the Newborn*, pp. 217–225. London, Baillière Tindall.

Department of Health (1993) Reviewing antenatal care. In (Expert Advisory Group, eds.) *Changing Childbirth*, pp. 19–22. London, HMSO.

Dimond B (1993) Stillbirths: Update. *Modern Midwife*, Mar: 14.

MacDonald G (1994) Personal communication, May 1994. MacDonald G, Co-ordinator, TAMBA (Twins and Multiple Birth Association) Bereavement Support Group, Box 30, Little Sutton, South Wirral L66 1TH.

Stillbirth (Definition) Act (1992). London, HMSO.

Terry PB (1990) Routine testing and prophylaxis. In (MH Hall, ed.) *Clinical Obstetrics and Gynaecology*, vol. 4, no. 1, pp. 25–43. London, Baillière Tindall.

Tew M (1995) The practices of attendants before birth. In (M Tew, ed.) *Safer Childbirth*, pp. 86–194. London, Chapman and Hall.

Acknowledgements

With thanks to my family, friends and colleagues who offered so much support in so many disguises, but especially to John, for learning more about the subject than I hope he ever needs to know.

Chapter One

Practical Issues Surrounding Care

Regardless of the nature of the perinatal loss, the gestation reached or the reason for death or termination, the issues surrounding the care given are similar for all types of death. Questions relating to the practical details such as where the delivery should take place or how the baby will look are faced by all staff. The following section is intended to address these issues and to provide some insight and, where possible, answers. What must be remembered is that each occasion is individual to the parents involved and assumptions about what is best for them must be avoided. Research into the area of perinatal loss is limited owing to the sensitivity of the subject matter. Mander noted that criticisms of care inevitably arise when mothers are asked to recount their experiences. She suggests that this may be because they are still trying to decide who is to blame for the death (Mander 1994).

DELIVERY SUITE VERSUS WARD AREA?

Trying to decide the best location in which to care for women whose babies have died or who are undergoing a termination of pregnancy is difficult: delivery suite versus gynaecology ward? antenatal ward versus postnatal ward? side-room versus main ward? Arguments exist for each area as the most suitable place. Often a decision is made, a policy is written and the reasons become lost in the mists of time; the staff become entrenched and pregnancies are dealt with in a certain way because that is the way it is done. Who is to challenge the status quo? The woman and her partner may never appreciate that an alternative may even exist. The health professional has to remain conscious of the choices available and to remember their position as the woman's advocate. It is to them she will turn for advice; if she fails to ask questions it is not acceptable to presume that she must know the answers. If she accepts what is suggested, the midwife, doctor or nurse has to ensure that the choices have been explained.

There is no correct answer to the dilemma. On the contrary, what is right for one couple may be totally unsuitable for the next (Hughes 1987). It is necessary for someone to take the lead and develop guidelines for good practice, taking into account the population served, the available resources within the unit and the staff involved. A standard for care must be formulated, audited at regular intervals and reviewed as necessary. Eighteen weeks gestation is often accepted as the rule for admission to the maternity unit rather than the gynaecology ward; a flexible approach to this guideline should be based on individual need.

The initial presentation may be to the Accident & Emergency Department. The medical staff will be called to review the client and make a diagnosis, following which the woman will be moved to the appropriate area. The middle of the night in a busy casualty unit is not the best environment in which to start a debate about the most suitable place to care for the woman. Her condition may prevent the client from joining in the discussion and a decision must often be made on her behalf. For a woman who finds herself in this situation the need to carry out medical treatment may be of paramount concern, especially if she is bleeding heavily or about to give birth. Where there is time to allow choice the mother's wishes should be determined. Staff need to ensure that the decision is not made without the couple being aware of the options – the noise of crying babies on a delivery suite may cause overwhelming distress to a bereaved couple; alternatively, they may be reassured by the sound of healthy babies. What is important is that the women are involved in the decision-making process about where they are nursed (Gohlish 1985; Hughes 1987; Henley and Kohner 1991; Mander 1991). Good intentions may prevail upon staff to avoid burdening the woman with mundane issues: this does not always achieve the desired result.

In the majority of situations the most appropriate location for the birth of the baby is the delivery suite. Here the availability of analgesia, including epidural anaesthesia, offers greater comfort for the mother. The area is designed to accommodate one-to-one care and privacy can be guaranteed in single rooms. If the pregnancy is being terminated because of maternal health, then close monitoring of her condition is permitted with ease of access to medical staff. Following the birth the mother may choose to remain in the delivery suite until she is discharged; alternatively, she may request a move to another ward until she is ready to leave. The concept of nursing a bereaved mother on an open ward housing healthy babies may be difficult for midwives to accept, but the reaction and care provided by other mothers may offer a lot of support for the woman without a cot beside here bed (Mander 1991). Having a home confinement for a stillbirth is not a choice many midwives or doctors would be particularly comfortable with. An induced labour would be difficult to achieve at home as the need for syntocinon augmentation would not be possible; there is also the potential need for an evacuation of the uterus following birth. If the labour starts at home and the woman chooses to remain in her comfortable, familiar surroundings, there is very little the midwife or GP can do to force the issue. If transfer to hospital becomes necessary during labour and the mother has previously refused to go to hospital, the midwife must inform the Supervisor of Midwives immediately for advice and assistance (UKCC 1994).

PLANNED ADMISSION TO THE DELIVERY SUITE

Once the decision to induce labour has been made, the staff need to co-ordinate the admission and liaise with their colleagues on the delivery suite. The couple should have the most influence over when the induction takes place, but they may need to be advised in the process. Factors to be taken into account include the request for an immediate postmortem and the number of other inductions occurring on the chosen day. Planning ahead also allows suitably experienced medical and midwifery staff to be on duty. This may include the Named Midwife, whose involvement can provide both continuity of care and reassurance during this traumatic time. As Mallinson explains:

> *A stillbirth can never be a joyful event, but sensitive, confident midwives can make labour and delivery a positive and successful experience for parents, and for themselves.*
> (Mallinson 1989)

The length of labour will vary according to the gestation and the parity of the individual. In general it is more difficult to achieve labour in a preterm pregnancy than induction after 38 weeks. However, the size of the preterm baby will allow delivery to occur before the cervix has dilated to 10 centimetres, which makes it hard to know when to prepare for the second stage. It is very possible that the labour will extend over more than one shift. It is essential that staff taking over the mother's care are fully briefed about information already discussed with the mother (Mander 1994).

The couple need to understand the process of induction and the estimated time involved. They should be encouraged to prepare for hours of waiting and advised to bring reading material and music to listen to. Although it will be hard for them to imagine being able to concentrate on anything other than the process in hand, there will be many hours of boredom and inactivity, particularly in the case of a therapeutic termination. Magazines and even television can help to pass the time without requiring serious concentration.

A companion is usually welcome and restrictions to visitors at this time should be discretionary. The majority of women will be clear about who they wish to see. Help from the staff may be necessary regarding visitors if the client is particularly young or very unsure of her own needs. Tremendous support can be provided by the visitors; the partner is usually present but circumstances may sometimes prevent this. An alternative may be a close friend or the client's mother. In some situations where the client has no-one in attendance the midwife's role as support becomes even more significant. The presence of an interpreter may be necessary and the staff should endeavour to obtain the services of someone for even a short period of time at the beginning of the induction. If the interpreter is unable to stay throughout the labour, they should arrange to return following the birth to assist in planning the client's discharge arrangements.

On the morning of admission the woman and her partner should be welcomed onto the delivery suite and introduced to the relevant members of staff. The couple should have time to familiarise themselves with the location of the bathroom, visitors' area and so forth. The partner may not wish to spend every moment in the delivery suite and advice about designated smoking areas and where to find refreshments should be provided. Once they have had the opportunity to get comfortable in the surroundings, the doctor may then visit the couple and repeat the information about the procedure for induction. This will vary according to local policy and the gestation reached.

In view of the potential need to perform an evacuation of the uterus following the delivery, it may be necessary for the women to restrict her oral intake. One of the difficulties with denying food or drink is not knowing how long the labour is going to last. Following discussion with the medical staff, particularly the anaesthetist, an agreement may be reached for a light diet to be given until the contractions begin. An intravenous infusion may then be commenced to avoid ketosis. Individual planning is necessary and it is unrealistic to adhere to a strict protocol. Guidelines for care may prove more appropriate.

Adequate provision of effective analgesia is an important issue for most women undergoing labour. The anticipation of giving birth to a dead baby is going to add a significant mental anguish to the actual physical pain, and any relief will often be welcomed by the mother. The midwife should seek advice from the anaesthetist for the most suitable analgesia to offer his or her client. For some an epidural will be the answer, while other women would prefer a more sedative effect to relief of the pain. Mander argues against the administration of large amounts of 'sedative', preferring for each mother to 'feel the amount of pain which she wants to feel' and to avoid total amnesia in favour of memories from the experience which will help her work through the grief (Mander 1994).

If vaginal pessaries have been used to induce labour, the woman may experience diarrhoea and/or pyrexia. As both side-effects can be distressing and further add to the feeling of loss of control, the midwife should warn the mother in advance about the possibility. If diarrhoea is present, the mother may be unable to distinguish the pressure from the baby and feel an urgent need to use the lavatory. The midwife should accompany the woman or ensure that she knows how to summon assistance.

Rupturing of the membranes is an area for debate and depends on individual hospital policy; concern exists around the potential risk of infection. The membranes may rupture spontaneously, but it is more common to deliver the baby in the amniotic sac.

LABOUR AND DELIVERY

The thrill of giving birth to a live, healthy baby is what makes the whole experience of labour worthwhile. Explaining to a woman that she is expected to endure hours of pain and physical discomfort for a dead baby can be viewed as cruelty beyond the worst form of torture. It is rare for anyone to consider labour as a positive experience in these circumstances.

The actual delivery of the baby will vary as for all cases. If the baby is preterm, very little effort may be required on the mother's part and the second stage may be rapid, occasionally taking everyone by surprise. Care should be taken when handling the baby. The use of an oxytocic agent will depend on the delivery. It is not unusual for the placenta to be retained and the umbilical cord may be friable and snap easily. If an evacuation of the uterus is required, this should be performed as soon as theatre time is available.

The more advanced the gestation, the more similar the second stage will be to the delivery of a live baby. The period of transition from the first to the second stage may cause as much distress as for a woman delivering a baby under normal conditions. The psychological barriers present during labour for a dead baby are many. These include the desire to get the process over with as quickly as possible and to end the nightmare. Despite this the mother may show an alarming reluctance to assist in any way with the birth. For the midwife who has supported the mother through hours of labour, there may now be complete confusion when he or she is faced with an uncooperative woman who appears, metaphorically speaking, to be crossing her legs in order not to give birth. The logic behind this rests in the reality factor – as long as the baby is *in utero* hope for that child can go on, the diagnosis may be wrong or a miracle may happen; but as soon as the baby is delivered the reality cannot be denied and no will-power in the world is going to change it, the mother will always have had a dead son or daughter.

When the baby is delivered the placenta should be attended to as for all deliveries. The use of an oxytocic agent should follow hospital policy and be administered with the mother's consent. Attention to the delivery of the placenta and membranes requires the same care as for all babies. If perineal trauma has occurred and sutures are required, the midwife or doctor should attend to this immediately. Adequate postnatal analgesia should be administered as required.

Choice of position for delivery of the baby should be left to the woman to adopt the way she feels most comfortable. The baby may be delivered onto her abdomen or however she desires. Discussing her intention to see and hold the baby in advance may be difficult, particularly because it will be hard for her to imagine how the baby will look. The midwife can do much to prepare her client but may also find it hard to describe the anatomical effect of certain abnormalities, for example anencephaly. A decision which is reached during the labour or beforehand should not be binding. The opportunity to reconsider her decision must be available and care must be taken by the professional not to influence the parents on the basis of personal belief. What a member of staff feels about a situation does not necessarily reflect the parents' feelings. Retaining control over the events which have overtaken them may be critical to the couple. Throughout the process of labour and delivery they should be consulted and have the opportunity to take part in decision making (Henley and Kohner 1991).

Handling of the dead baby should be performed with the same tenderness reserved for the living. The baby should be wrapped in suitable baby clothes as soon as possible and may require a bath before being presented to the parents. Even when the baby is alive, some parents find it distressing to see their baby covered in liquor and blood. The presence of the cot in the delivery room may have been upsetting to the couple and it may have been removed before labour commenced. The purpose of a cot is to provide a resting place for a baby, something which is still required when the baby is dead; the hospital may have a special Moses-style basket specifically for this purpose or use a general cot. The importance of communication with the parents continues to be essential in deciding this issue. Their appreciation of the need to nurse their baby in a suitable place and their personal wishes should be adhered to. Removing all evidence of the baby's needs may be to deny the existence of the child (Mander 1994).

If the parents have decided against holding the baby immediately, they should be aware of where he or she is and perhaps will be happy to have the cot next to the bed. For the couple who find themselves in this unfamiliar environment it may be very difficult to ask questions or to express their real desires. The midwife must be observant for hidden messages or signals in the behaviour and body language of the woman and her partner. It may be that the couple have different needs and wishes but that each is unable to voice them for fear of upsetting the other. Continuity of carer will help to overcome some of these issues and enhance the trust which the couple place in the team who are caring for them. One of the fears couples have is not knowing what the baby will look like. The discovery of an abnormality with a terrifying name may conjure up images of horror. This may present a quandary for the midwife who wishes to encourage the couple to overcome their fears although they may have no desire to see the baby themselves. Delicate negotiation is required, enabling the parents to revisit the decision in the future by giving them information about how long the baby will be available for viewing before the postmortem or burial. If the parents do choose to see the baby, the presentation should be handled sensitively. Care should be taken to cover affected parts of the body (such as using a hat to cover an anencephalic baby's skull) for the initial viewing. The body can then be uncovered slowly at a pace comfortable for the parents. Live babies are always seen naked by the couple until the concern for warmth dictates the need to dress the baby. It is important that the couple who have a dead baby have the opportunity to see all of him or her. They need to see for themselves the sex of the baby and the number of toes on each foot. Attention can be focused on the tiny aspects of the baby such as the fingernails, which are usually perfect, or the colour of the hair. On close inspection family resemblances may be apparent to the couple. To be able to say 'He looked like you' may be very healing in the months ahead. One look may not be enough, live babies are placed with the mother to care for and to bond with in her own time so that she can observe and get to know her baby. When the baby is dead the amount of time the couple spend with their child is controlled by the staff and may depend on the midwife's personal view of what is acceptable. Conditions in a hot delivery suite are not conducive to prolonged time in a warm room but this should not prevent the parents having access to their child; they may need to visit the hospital mortuary to continue their time with the baby.

Viewing the baby may be very important to other members of the family. Siblings can be involved in a very positive way when a baby has died, particularly as children can have clear ideas about life and death. Much depends on their age and the previous information the children have received. Denying them access to the reality of the situation may not be in their best interest for the future. With care and support the children may be able to see and hold their brother or sister. Photographs can be taken to record the event; the inclusion of the dead baby in a family photograph may sound macabre to some parents, but the reality is that the baby will always have been a member of that family. Grandparents may also choose to see their grandchild and to be photographed holding the baby (Henley and Kohner, 1991; Stewart and Dent 1994).

With the exception of babies who are immediately transferred to the neonatal unit it is routine for midwives to check all babies following delivery. Parents are always keen to know details about their son or daughter, generally asking for the weight before the umbilical cord has been severed. The initial check is a top to toe examination of the newborn, taking into account deviations from the norm such as a extra digit or a tongue tie which are then referred to the paediatrician. When the baby is born dead the midwife should still carry out the check. The parents may already have consented to a postmortem, but the pathologist will still require information from the delivery such as the birthweight. For the parents it is important to know facts about their child, and the information should be written down, possibly on a cot card, and given to them to keep.

Photographs should be taken as soon as possible following the delivery (Mallinson 1989), regardless of whether the couple wish to have the photographs or not. It is much better to store unwanted photographs which are never claimed than not to have any when the parents change their mind. For this reason it is necessary that the couple know that the photographs are available for as long as the notes are stored. Taking photographs of the dead baby has become more acceptable. Attention to detail such as the background and the angle of the baby is now routine. Generally a Polaroid camera is used which provides instant images of the baby. Unfortunately, the print tends to fade over the years, although this can be overcome by advising the parents to take it to a professional photographer and have a long-term copy made. The alternative is to take a roll of 24 or 36 shots on an instamatic camera and give the film to the parents to have developed when they are ready (Stewart and Dent 1994). Photographs of the parents holding the baby make a good keepsake, and other children or grandparents may also be included. The important part is to offer choice to the couple.

Photographs create memories of the baby who has been lost. There are very few tangible mementos which staff can provide. The importance of having evidence of the baby's existence has been revealed time and again (Lewis 1982; Mallinson 1989; Forrest 1991; Henley and Kohner 1991; Stewart and Dent 1994; Kohner and Henley 1991). Recognition of the deceased is an important factor in the mourning process. Memorial services are held in memory of the lifetime achievement of the dead; a stillborn baby has been denied the opportunity to provide memories beyond the womb, so every tiny fragment of the baby's short existence is precious.

Keeping a lock of hair may be possible. Culturally there may be some objection to this, so it is wise for the midwife to enquire first (Stewart and Dent 1994). Babies' hair is downy and may need to be shaved rather than cut from the head. Folding the hair into tissue paper for safe keeping will be necessary until the parents decide what to do with it.

Footprints and handprints are unique to the baby and may easily be obtained using an inkpad. Small cards such as those used for birth announcements can be used as the base. The earlier the gestation the more fragile the skin will be and, in the case of a baby who has been dead *in utero* for some days, skin maceration may have occurred, making the imprint difficult. The midwife should be careful when holding the foot and must wipe the ink off afterwards.

If the head circumference or the length of the baby have been measured, the parents can be given the tape measure as a memento. Recordings of the measurements can be duplicated for the couple.

One of the key indicators of success as defined by the Expert Maternity Group in *Changing Childbirth* (Department of Health 1993) is that women carry their own casenotes throughout pregnancy. In a great many units this is already standard practice and women are becoming accustomed to the layout and terminology found within the notes. In many hospitals, planning teams of midwives and obstetricians have worked together to make the notes more user friendly. The same language and medicalisation problems exist with regard to the information given to couples following a perinatal death. With some revision, all documentation with respect to the baby and its care could be photocopied and given to the parents. Translation of the medical terminology into plain English would be helpful to the parents. Efforts have been made in Western Australia to demedicalise the process of consent to postmortem examination and a plain-language report is now given in place of the full technical report (Knowles 1994).

Religion may be important to the parents and staff need to assist them in contacting the necessary minister. Awareness of particular religious beliefs and expectations concerning the death of someone are necessary in providing quality care. For larger cities where communities gather in the same locality, such as the Muslim population in the East End of London, the religious needs of the woman may be readily catered for. The religious representation in the local hospital providing medical services to the East End includes an Imam who is available to provide information and advice for staff.

Transfer of the baby to the mortuary is generally a portering responsibility. A suitable container should be used and the parents should be aware that the baby has been moved. All documentation necessary to accompany the baby should be completed and included at the time of transfer. Clear indication regarding consent to the postmortem should be given to avoid confusion and the possible release of a baby for burial before the examination is carried out. The mortuary will need to know if the parents are still undecided and will then await further instruction from the ward.

Communication is the key to the successful management of the process following the delivery of a dead baby. Clear documentation in the casenotes will help future discussions with the parents, particularly if they have questions about the labour or delivery. Before going off duty each midwife must ensure that his or her records are up to date and that all necessary information regarding the woman has been handed over to the oncoming staff.

Certain information may need to be repeated for the benefit of the bereaved mother. During the course of labour and birth she will have received a large amount of information, only some of which she can retain. The couple who were anticipating a live birth until the moment of delivery will be particularly vulnerable at this point and unable to focus on anything other than the devastating event which has just overtaken them. The more senior members of staff have a duty to support less-experienced colleagues who are caring for the couple.

Postnatal care for the bereaved mother must acknowledge that she will undergo the same physical process as women with a livebirth. Expectations of what is likely to happen on which day, such as the breastmilk 'coming in' should not take her by surprise. Anticipation of such a physiological process with an understanding of why it has occurred and how it should be managed will help the women to accept the changes. The use of bromocriptine tablets to stem the production of breastmilk may not always be of great value. When the course of oral medication has been completed there is a possibility that the milk will be produced anyway, thereby providing a late reminder of the loss. Information regarding bromocriptine should be given to the woman and she should be allowed to decide whether or not to take it.

During the postnatal period the woman may continue to be nursed in the delivery suite; often this depends on the type of delivery and the proposed length of stay, plus the suitability of the room. A dedicated bereavement room would be the optimum choice, particularly as the design usually takes into account the partner's needs, but this is not always available. In certain circumstances it may be possible for the mother to leave hospital within a few hours of the birth. If so, then the vital links will be the midwife who cares for her at home and the woman's GP.

There is the possibility that the woman will have undergone a caesarean section and will need to stay in hospital longer for postoperative care which may necessitate a transfer to the postnatal ward. In a larger ward area the woman is more exposed and the potential for someone to say the wrong thing is greater. Porters are often involved in the transferring of women to the wards. Usually the baby accompanies the mother and the porter may not be conscious of the different circumstances. Confidentiality is a key issue in the care of women and the midwife is unlikely to be in a position to warn the porter to proceed with caution. Potentially embarrassing situations can occur at any time and the midwife needs to be adept at handling them. This is easier said than done: in the scenario described the mother may react well and answer questions about her baby without becoming visibly distressed; alternatively, she may break down and the porter will be upset to have unwittingly caused distress. There is little the midwife can do at this time other than comfort the woman. Later she can contact the porter and discuss the issue with him or her, offering reassurance that the woman will be fine and that crying is not harmful and that there will be no long-term effects.

If the woman is transferred to another ward area, she should be offered a single room. Her preference may be to mix with the other postnatal women in the general ward area. If so, the midwife should ensure that the woman appreciates the implications of sharing a ward. Natural curiosity and a desire to share in the happy event may inspire questions about her absent baby. In today's society babies are not expected to die and, although most women would acknowledge that it can happen, they will not expect to meet someone in the hospital whose baby has died. From their perspective it may make life very uncomfortable, particularly if the bereaved mother is visibly upset in their presence. It takes a strong woman to be surrounded by healthy babies and happy families when she has given birth to a dead baby. So is it wise to allow women the option of being in the ward? In the absence of research evidence, opinions will continue to vary on this subject. At the end of the day the choice should be left to the woman.

The pregnancy may have involved more than one baby and the mother may, in fact, have a surviving neonate to nurse. To the other postnatal mothers she will appear perfectly normal as a woman with a child, the real circumstances hidden by the healthy baby. In addition, this mother presents a combination of grief and relief. Her reaction may be very mixed and present a totally different challenge to staff. Here is a woman with a very real reminder of exactly what she has lost. Her breastmilk will be required and time will be taken up in caring for the surviving baby while thinking about funeral arrangements and trying to mourn.

The alternative to the main ward is usually a side-room, which may achieve the opposite effect and totally isolate the woman. Owing to their own inability to deal with the mother's grief, staff may avoid the room except when attending to essential nursing duties. Allocating time in a busy postnatal ward to talk to a bereaved mother can be difficult in many situations. Often, even when the staff are able to deal with the mother's grief, it is not the right moment for her (Mander 1994).

On arrival to the postnatal ward the usual routine of welcome and introduction by the midwife should follow. Depending on her condition and mobility the mother should be aware of the ward layout and know how to find the bathroom and lavatory. Meals may be taken with the other women in the dining room or by her bedside. Much will depend on her physical condition and mental state. Perinatal death creates a situation where a person is recently bereaved and, at the same time, recovering from medical care and possibly surgery. During the postnatal period the woman has to overcome the same physical changes as those with healthy babies. It is important that some acknowledgement is made of her status within the ward environment – an identified symbol may be used such as the SANDS teardrop sticker. The sticker or symbol is attached to the room door and to the casenotes in order to avoid causing upset through ignorance.

DOCUMENTATION

Record keeping is recognised within the Midwives' Rules as of paramount importance in the care of all women and babies:

> *(1) A practising midwife shall keep as contemporaneously as is reasonable detailed records of observations, care given and medicine or other forms of pain relief administered by her to all mothers and babies.*
>
> Rule 42
> (UKCC 1993)

The casenotes should contain a clear account of the care throughout labour and delivery. Each member of staff involved in the case is responsible for documenting their care and for communicating with colleagues. Provided that the woman has booked for antenatal care, she will have a set of maternity casenotes; these should be used in all situations where the woman is cared for within the maternity department. Different arrangements may apply on the gynaecology ward and local policy may affect the detailed aspects of some casenotes.

The present climate of computerised documentation does not significantly reduce the amount of paperwork involved in perinatal loss. Fears that the communication systems will break down necessitate the creation of checklists. But what do they achieve? Is our care better because of them? Or do they depersonalise the process? Forrest suggests they are used as *aides-mémoire* rather than a replacement for personalised, compassionate contact with staff (Forrest 1991). Examples of checklists can be found in most maternity units, but owing to the variation in procedures and guidelines surrounding perinatal loss it would be impossible to design a universal form. The ideal checklist would provide sufficient information to ensure continuity of care without unnecessary duplication. It is important to avoid the 'cookbook' approach to providing care (Mander 1994). One advantage of a checklist is that it can be initiated at the onset of care; for example, a woman experiencing a spontaneous abortion may transfer through the accident and emergency department, the operating theatre and eventually the gynaecology ward. During the process she may encounter a number of nurses and doctors who provide her with some information: the checklist can be used to document this and build up a picture to enable the ward staff to meet her outstanding needs (Ryan et al 1991). Alternatively, the checklist can be used at shift changeover to inform staff of what has been discussed. Typically the checklist includes areas such as who informed the parents of the baby's death; which members of the medical staff were informed; was consent for postmortem obtained; did the parents view the baby and were photographs taken; was a religious leader involved; has an entry been recorded in the Book of Remembrance; were funeral arrangements discussed; has an appointment been made for the postnatal follow-up; and so on. Some may include the necessary blood tests which are required from the mother and particular specimens from the baby.

A checklist will provide staff with the chance to see at a glance what has been done and what is outstanding. It is not possible to achieve everything immediately and it may be days before decisions are made about funerals or postmortems. Certain documentation is required to be completed 'contemporaneously' – existing or occurring at the same time according to the Oxford English Dictionary. The casenotes are an ongoing account of the woman's condition and progress, the information contained within them must be factual, written at the time and a true record of events. Information entered onto a computerised casenote system must be checked by the midwife or doctor to ensure that it is accurate.

A birth notification will be required for all babies born after 24 weeks gestation or less if signs of life were present. The information entered onto the form must be provided by a midwife who examined the baby and can confirm that it is correct. Prior to 24 weeks there is no legal requirement to record the baby's birth unless he or she was a live birth.

Consent to postmortem and chromosome studies should always be requested after perinatal death; these may provide invaluable information about the cause of death, not only helping parents with their grief but also assisting with the planning of future pregnancies (Forrest 1991). The consent form is not a legal requirement before a postmortem can be carried out, but it is good practice and few hospitals would embark on the examination if the parents expressed a negative view. In situations where the pregnancy is being terminated for an abnormality, the postmortem will have been mentioned and the parents given some idea of the process involved. They may have questions about the damage, as they see it, to their baby and may need reassurance about being able to view the baby afterwards. Once the consent is given the parents hold high hopes of the results. It is important that they receive the information in a form which they can understand, preferably by verbal account from a senior doctor at the postnatal follow-up appointment.

A certificate of stillbirth is required for all babies born after 24 weeks gestation who did not have any signs of life following complete expulsion from the mother. The attending medical practitioner has a statutory duty to issue a certificate; if a doctor is unavailable a midwife may complete the certificate if she or he was present for the delivery of the stillbirth or examined the baby afterwards. As far as possible the cause of death and the estimated duration of the pregnancy should be entered (UKCC 1994, p. 25).

In the case of a pre-viable fetus who has not shown signs of life following delivery before 24 weeks, a certificate is not a legal requirement. A certificate may be issued for two reasons; firstly it provides the parents with an acknowledgement that their baby existed and, secondly, the parents may wish to arrange a private funeral and the hospital and the funeral director will require some formal paperwork in order to get the baby released from the hospital mortuary. The usual process is for the deceased to be registered and a death certificate issued; the family then give this form to the undertaker, who exchanges it for the appropriate body from the mortuary. In the case of a pre-viable baby, no such formal documentation exists, therefore a local agreement with the hospital is required to create an acceptable certificate. Hospital notepaper with letterhead should be used, containing the relevant information of the baby's sex, date of birth/death and the mother's details. The paper must be signed by a registered midwife or doctor.

If the baby was born alive and subsequently died, a death certificate will be issued by a medical practitioner who was present. The certificate must be taken to the Registrar and the baby recorded as a live birth and then a death. In this case a death certificate will then be given and forwarded to the funeral director. (See Appendix 1A.)

Recording details of the child who has died in a Book of Remembrance can be very important to parents. Access to a book of this nature can be seen as evidence of the hospital's recognition for the life which has been lost. Parents have the opportunity to put their feelings into print as a permanent reminder of their baby. The form of the Book of Remembrance varies from hospital to hospital, some being more sophisticated than others but all fulfilling the same need. A professionally bound book with expert calligraphy skills available to make the entries is very aesthetically pleasing, but equally effective and significant may be a notebook with handwritten entries by the relatives.

The *Changing Childbirth* document includes the objective that midwives and GPs work together in the best interests of the woman (Department of Health 1993). Communication between the two groups is vital for continuity of care to the vulnerable mother whose baby has died. The discharge summary must be completed in the appropriate form for the hospital. Local policy may dictate that the information is supported by telephone contact. Allowing the woman to go home without informing her GP puts her at potential risk of fragmented care. Regardless of whether he or she was involved in the antenatal care, the GP should have been told the outcome of the pregnancy, particularly if they were anticipating carrying out the baby check. Staff must plan ahead to avoid potentially embarrassing and distressing situations.

Informing the antenatal clinic is important as the woman will not attend any outstanding appointments. This may lead to her receiving a telephone call or letter about her non-attendance, either of which can be distressing on both sides.

Audit of clinical practice is becoming an increasingly familiar concept within the maternity services. Every 3 years the Confidential Enquiry into Maternal Deaths is published. The audit includes recommendations for improvement in clinical practice to reduce the number of deaths as much as possible (Kirkup 1990). The monitoring of perinatal deaths has been taking place in Scotland since 1983, incorporated into the data collection system which monitors maternal and child health in Scotland (McIlwaine et al 1985). The Confidential Enquiry into Stillbirths and Deaths in Infancy (CESDI) commenced in England, Wales and Northern Ireland in 1993. Its aim was to identify ways to prevent the number of deaths which occur, acknowledging that the percentage of perinatal deaths has declined over the last thirty years to 7.6 per 1000 births in 1993 (Department of Health 1995).

The process of audit involves gathering information on all deaths within the agreed criteria; in the case of CESDI a National Advisory Body was introduced to consider data from 20 weeks gestation to the end of the first year of life. Data collection commenced on 1 January 1993. The terms of reference for the National Advisory Body as set out in March 1992 are

> *To guide, support, oversee and co-ordinate the Confidential Enquiry into Stillbirths and Deaths in Infancy, nationwide; to receive, report on and disseminate the findings; and to make recommendations for action. The National Advisory Body will make an annual report to the Ministers.*
>
> (Department of Health 1995)

In Scotland the first perinatal audit was undertaken as a retrospective research study in 1977. The casenotes of each death were observed and the results from the study were analysed the following year and made available to each division of obstetrics. By 1982 all obstetricians were providing information on deaths which occurred in their hospital or district (McIlwaine et al 1985).

As with all types of clinical audit, staff participation is critical. It is easy to acknowledge the importance of confidential enquiries when the paperwork involves such a tiny number as with maternal mortality. In the case of perinatal loss this is more difficult as there are more deaths to report on; the fact that most hospitals conduct a regular audit meeting into perinatal morbidity and/or mortality indicates recognition of the importance of learning what we can from these deaths. Identifying a named person to take responsibility for the collection of information makes the process easier, although this does not exclude others from participating or taking responsibility.

DISCHARGE

Discharge from hospital should be dependent on the woman's medical and psychological condition. If a physical problem is identified, the doctor should be informed and should prescribe the necessary treatment. It may be difficult for a woman to come to terms with the recognition her body is going to behave as though she has given birth to a live baby. Reassurance from the staff will help her to accept this; for continuity of care it is important that all communication or concerns the mother has expressed are passed on to the next midwife or doctor, including how they were dealt with to date.

Preparation for home should allow time for the couple to talk about their fears. In some instances the woman may not want to return to the outside world where everything waits for her baby; she may find reasons to remain in hospital and avoid the reality of an empty nursery or cot for as long as possible. It may be that concerned friends or relatives have removed all evidence of preparation for the baby before she returns; this may be the correct approach for some women, but it is an area for debate. Other women may want to take time putting the items away themselves as a way of saying goodbye to their baby. Alternatively, some women want to be discharged as quickly as possible following delivery of the baby because the hospital serves as a reminder of what they have lost and they want to return to familiar surroundings. The comforts of home may become very precious at this time, particularly if there are other children to consider. Staff should attempt to meet the woman's needs and enable her to make the right decision for herself.

Following the death of a baby the immediate care focuses on the woman's physical health and the couple's emotional state. Visitors are usually prepared for the news and it is rare for the hospitalised woman to have to tell anyone what has happened. This situation changes on discharge: while the immediate family and friends and staff are aware, neighbours may not be. This can lead to emotional confrontations where the woman is taken by surprise when she ventures to the corner shop and is greeted with congratulations because she is obviously no longer pregnant.

If the pregnancy has ended in a spontaneous abortion before the woman has commenced maternity leave, she may require a medical certificate of sickness. The GP or hospital doctor can provide this. Difficulties in returning to work may depend on the nature of the job and the relationship with colleagues; the prospect of life continuing as normal may be very alien to the couple who have just experienced the loss of their baby. Time will inevitably help the adjustment, but caution against rushing the process is advisable.

Family planning advice needs to be given in a sensitive and caring manner. Avoiding an unplanned pregnancy and preparing for the future are very important aspects of the puerperium. The woman should be encouraged to talk about this with her partner and to seek further advice and support if necessary from her GP.

Talking about the loss will help the couple to come to terms with the reality of it. However, this may be difficult depending on their cultural beliefs, their relationship with each other, the way in which they have handled the grieving process and a multitude of other factors. Outside support from organisations such as the Stillbirth and Neonatal Death Society (SANDS), Support After Termination for Abnormality (SATFA) and the Miscarriage Association can be sought as appropriate. Most of these organisations are dependent on voluntary carers or befrienders who are prepared to offer support in group settings or by telephone. Access is usually left to the individual as the purpose is to provide help when she and her partner are ready for it. Referral by a concerned midwife or doctor may be too soon or may make the woman feel the process to be medically led. The issues regarding counselling for bereaved couples and their families are covered in Chapter 2.

For the postnatal check at six weeks the woman may attend her GP or return to the hospital and see the obstetrician. A special clinic may have been set up for these couples as the visit provides the opportunity to discuss the case, to answer questions and to plan for the future. If a postmortem examination has been performed, the results should be available by this time. The alternative venue would be the gynaecology clinic, but it will be necessary to ensure that the appointment is not rushed as there will be much to talk about. The midwife or nurse who cared for the woman in labour may wish to be present and provide continuity. Discussing future pregnancies may be very important as it may be advisable for the couple to see a geneticist or have prenatal screening. If the loss of the baby was unexplained, they will need reassurance about the potential success of the next pregnancy.

If the couple are unhappy in any way with the care which they received they should be encouraged to express this. A simple explanation may clear up a misunderstanding; alternatively, there may be valuable lessons to be learned from hearing about the individual experience.

REFERENCES

Department of Health (1993) Reviewing antenatal care. In (Expert Maternity Group, eds) *Changing Childbirth*, pp 19–22. London, HMSO.

Department of Health (1995) *Confidential Enquiry into Stillbirth and Deaths in Infancy* Part 1. London, HMSO.

Forrest GC (1991) Coping after stillbirth. *Maternal and Child Health* **31**: 394–398.

Gohlish MC (1985) Stillbirth. *Midwife, Health Visitor and Community Nurse* **21**: 16–22.

Henley A & Kohner N (1991) *Hospital Care: Guidelines for Professionals*, pp. 18–32. London, SANDS.

Hughes P (1987) The management of bereaved mothers: What is best? *Midwives Chronicle and Nursing Notes* Aug.: 226–229.

Kirkup W (1990) Perinatal audit: Does confidential enquiry have a place? *British Journal of Obstetrics and Gynaecology* **97**: 371–373.

Knowles S (1994) A passage through grief: The Western Australia Rural Pregnancy Loss Team. *British Medical Journal* **309**: 1705–1708.

Kohner N & Henley A (1991) Experiences in hospital. In *When a Baby Dies*, pp 47–109. London, SANDS.

Lewis H (1982) Coping with stillbirth. *New Society* Apr.: 54.

Mallinson G (1989) When a baby dies. *Nursing Times* **85**: 31–34.

Mander R (1991) Midwifery care of the grieving mother: How the decisions are made. *Midwifery* **7**: 133–142.

Mander R (1994) Caring for the grieving mother. In (R Mander, ed.) *Loss and Bereavement in Childbearing*, pp 56–74. Oxford, Blackwell Scientific Publications.

McIlwaine GM, Dunn FH, Howat RC, Smalls M, Wyllie MM & McNaughton MC (1985) A routine system for monitoring perinatal deaths in Scotland. *British Journal of Obstetrics and Gynaecology* **92**: 9–13.

PRACTICAL ISSUES
– Discharge

Ryan PF, Côte-Arsenault D & Sugarman LL (1991) Facilitating care after perinatal loss: A comprehensive checklist. *Journal of Obstetrics, Gynaecology and Neonatal Nursing*, Sept.: 385–388.

Stewart A & Dent A (1994) Lost beginnings: When a pregnancy ends before birth. In (A Stewart & A Dent, eds) *At a Loss*, pp 13–50. London, Baillière Tindall.

UKCC (1993) Responsibility and sphere of practice. In *Midwives' Rules*, Section 40. United Kingdom Central Council for Nurses, Midwives and Health Visitors.

UKCC (1994) Supervisor of midwives. In *The Midwives' Code of Practice*, Rule 44. United Kingdom Central Council for Nurses, Midwives and Health Visitors.

APPENDIX 1A: REGISTRATION PROCEDURE

There is a legal obligation to record the baby's existence in the following circumstances.

England and Wales

A livebirth or a stillbirth must be registered within 42 days. The registration must take place in the registration district in which the death occurred, which may not be the district in which the parents live. The registrar may attend the woman in hospital to register the baby but this will depend on individual arrangements with the local office. The baby will be registered in the name of the married couple or that of the mother. If the couple are unmarried, the father may not register the baby in his name without the mother being in attendance.

Scotland

A birth or a stillbirth should be registered within 21 days by a primary informant. In the case of a child born to parents who are married to each other, the primary informant is either the mother or the father. If the parents are not married to each other, the mother is the primary informant. The name of the father may only be entered in the birth entry provided:

- he attends the registrar's office with the mother and they both sign the birth or stillbirth entry;

or

- there is produced to the registrar at the time of the registration (a) a declaration on Form 26 naming the father and signed by the mother in the registrar's presence, and (b) a statutory declaration acknowledging paternity signed by the father before a Justice of the Peace or a Notary Public. In this case the mother would sign the entry;

or

• there is produced to the registrar (a) a declaration on Form 27 acknowledging paternity which is signed by the father in the registrar's presence, and (b) a statutory declaration naming the father and signed by the mother before a Justice of the Peace or a Notary Public. In this case the father would sign the entry.

The appropriate forms are available in the office of the registrar in Scotland and can be asked for by number.

In some circumstances, for example if the primary informant is seriously ill, a secondary informant may be acceptable to the registrar to register the birth or stillbirth. A secondary informant may be one of the following:

(i)   a relative of either parent having knowledge of the birth or stillbirth;
(ii) the occupier of the premises in which the child was born;
(iii) any person present at the birth.

Deaths should be registered within 8 days by a qualified informant. The qualified informants to a death are as follows:

(i) any relative of the deceased;
(ii) any person present at the death.

If the baby's parents are not married to each other, the father's particulars can be entered in the death entry if known.

The Registration of Births, Deaths and Marriages (Scotland) Act 1965 requires that a medical practitioner shall, within 7 days after the death, transmit the Medical Certificate of Cause of Death to the person who is a qualified informant to the death, or to the registrar.

In the case of a stillbirth, a Certificate of Stillbirth should be issued by the medical practitioner or midwife who was present at the birth or who examined the baby (General Register Office for Scotland, New Register House, Edinburgh, EH1 3YT).

Northern Ireland

The legal requirement is again to register the baby within 42 days of the birth. In the case of a neonatal death the registration must occur within 5 days from the date of occurrence, except where the case has been referred to the Coroner. The 5-day period may be extended to 14 if the registrar is notified in writing of the death and supplied with a medical certificate of the cause.

The occupation of the father may be required in addition to his full name and date of birth. If the parents are not married, the mother's full name and date of birth will also be required. The father of the baby cannot register his child out of wedlock unless the mother is present. If neither parent is able to register the baby, an alternative may be:

(i)   a grandparent, aunt or uncle who has knowledge of the birth;
(ii)   the occupier of the premises in which the baby was born;
(iii) any person present at the birth.

A stillbirth certificate is required for all babies.

If the baby is born in a maternity hospital, he or she may be registered with the District Registrar, who attends on certain days (General Register Office for Northern Ireland, Oxford House, 49–55 Chichester Street, Belfast BT1 4HL).

In all situations the registrar will require information about the baby; the date of birth and death (if different), the cause of death if known (the certificate from the doctor or midwife will inform the registrar if a postmortem is being performed), and the baby's full name. The parents should be aware that they will only be able to register the baby's forename on this first occasion.

FURTHER READING

Kohner N (1985) The Report of the Joint Royal College of Midwives/ Health Education Council Workshop held in October 1994. In *Midwives and Stillbirths*. London, Health Education Council.

Chapter Two

Counselling

Response to the death of a loved one can be extremely varied depending on the relationship with the deceased. For the bereaved the grieving process is a gradual progression through a time of mourning and deep sorrow as memories of the dead person replace their actual presence. The loss of a baby before delivery does not allow memories to be created; there is very little tangible evidence of the existence of the life which has ended and the prospective parents are denied the opportunity to develop a firm relationship with their child. In all circumstances the grieving process may alter to a complicated course for which professional help is required. In the case of perinatal loss the grieving process is remarkably uncharted territory and there are few markers for the health professional to detect a deterioration in the bereaved mother. A first step is for the midwife, nurse or doctor to recognise that the mother has sustained a real loss (Worden 1992).

Priorities of care may indicate that the physical effect on the woman requires immediate care and attention, but the psychological impact must not be ignored. The tendency on the part of the medical and nursing staff to overlook the need for counselling may be related to their own ability to deal with the death. The purpose of this chapter is to consider those vital hours around the time of delivery and in the immediate postnatal period when professional counselling help may not be available and the untrained doctor, nurse or midwife has to fulfil the role. Consideration is given to the grieving process and the various responses to death.

GRIEF

Grief is a lonely, isolating emotion. According to Worden, grief may be uncomplicated or complicated (Worden 1992). In the majority of situations grief is uncomplicated and the bereaved moves through a process of mourning which may be divided into stages (Kubler-Ross 1992), phases (Parkes 1970) or tasks (Worden

1992) until life resumes a more familiar pattern. An interruption to the grieving process may lead to a more complicated pattern which can take years to resolve but, owing to the individualised nature of grief, it can be difficult to identify the difference.

> *Death is still a fearful, frightening happening and the fear of death is a universal fear ...*
>
> (Kubler-Ross 1992)

Grief can manifest itself through intense and diverse feelings: acute reactions may bring on physical sensations such as tightness in the chest, hollowness in the stomach and muscle weakness. In the process of uncomplicated grief the individual would be expected to experience some extremes of feelings. Worden (1992) listed commonly found emotions:

shock	*numbness*
loneliness	*anger*
helplessness	*anxiety*
yearning	*emancipation*
guilt	*self-reproach*
sadness	*relief*
fatigue	

Example: **An intrauterine death at 38 weeks gestation**
At a routine antenatal visit the midwife is unable to auscultate the fetal heart and refers the client to the obstetrician. For the woman *shock* is replaced by *numbness* as the death is confirmed by an ultrasound scan. Waiting for her partner to arrive, she experiences intense feelings of *loneliness*. She may be *angry* with the staff for not predicting the outcome while feeling *helpless* at losing control of the situation. There is *anxiety* at the prospect of experiencing labour and a deep *yearning* for the baby inside. Discussion with the medical staff regarding inducing the labour may result in a desire for *emancipation* from carrying this dead baby, to be quickly replaced by *guilt* and *self-reproach*. The events in general can lead to a feeling of extreme *sadness* with intense *relief* when the delivery is over. Eventually *fatigue* replaces the conflicting emotions, leaving a desire to sleep it all away.

In situations of terminal illness some preparation for grief is possible. The death of a baby before delivery tends to be unexpected and allows little preparation time (Department of Health 1994). The pregnant woman may consider the developing baby to be an extension of herself and strong bonds can be forged during the long gestation period, a one-sided attachment to the baby, to whom she talks, sings and plays music. Encouragement to plan families can lead to a loss of control when the pregnancy ends in death.

Theut found that the degree of grief felt depended on the gestation reached, suggesting that an attachment to the developing baby may influence the loss felt (Theut et al 1989). In the case of a fetal abnormality the woman acquires time to consider the outcome, but a decision regarding the continuation of the pregnancy is usually required.

Of all life events having and raising children are among the most significant (Kohn and Moffitt 1994). Taken for granted, the discovery that pregnancy is not an easy path to tread can provide deep shock for couples who are infertile or unable to carry the pregnancy to a viable stage.

Loss can present itself in many guises, not all of them sad. The loss of a sister through marriage tends to mean an addition to the family and the original sibling relationship may be lost (Stewart and Dent 1994). Learning how to adapt to different types of loss varies according to the age of the individual and the support mechanisms in place. For women who experience the loss of a baby at birth there may be a restricted amount of support as close friends and family are unaccustomed to bereavement of this sort.

THE MOURNING PROCESS

Various stages, phases or tasks have been identified through working with the dying and bereaved (Parkes 1970; Kubler-Ross 1992; Worden 1992). Reaction to a fetal death may strongly resemble that to the death of an adult or child. The effect may be visible in the extended family and friends who have been involved in the pregnancy and have shared the plans for the future of this particular baby. There are no definite rules to follow in the mourning process; stages may be reached at a different pace and some may be passed by completely. At the centre of the range of feelings is the principle that the bereaved is trying to come to terms with a major life experience (Kennedy and Charles 1991). The following are the most commonly identified reactions.

Denial

The Victorian attitude to death and infant mortality was a more accepting one than that of society today. Advances in medical sciences and social circumstances have left the developed world with high and often unreal expectations of childbirth. Despite the facts that 1 in 5 first pregnancies end in spontaneous abortion or that the perinatal mortality rate is 8.6 per 1000 births, it remains difficult to talk about the possibility of an unsuccessful outcome (Department of Health 1994). Mander likens it to the Victorian attitude towards sex, suggesting that the current emphasis is on young, healthy, sexually active people despite the increasing number of elderly (Mander 1994).

A reaction of total denial to the news that the baby is dead is not uncommon. The denial may last throughout the labour and delivery. Even when the mother has held the baby in her arms she may still talk as though the child were alive. Although, to the staff caring for her, denial of this nature may cause alarm, it is important to allow her space to express her grief. Denying the death may be the first personal stage in a situation which is too overwhelming to accept. An over-reaction by staff at this point may cause the mourning to become complicated. The benefit of a Named Midwife in this situation is that the relationship has existed for sufficient time to allow the midwife to know the mother and her response to the pregnancy. If the midwife has walked in 'cold' to care for this woman in labour, he or she has to build up that relationship in the worst moments. Help can be sought from other family members or a religious person who is acceptable to the woman.

For some couples it is sufficient to deny the death until the point of delivery; when the baby is in their arms they can begin to accept what they have lost. To the mother and her partner many hopes and dreams will have died with the heartbeat, including the opportunity to parent this child.

There may be underlying reasons to the denial, one partner may have experienced the death of someone close in the past, and the association may be too difficult to confront. It may be that the mother or partner experienced ambivalent feelings towards the pregnancy earlier on and is using denial to avoid feelings of guilt.

The staff may also react to the news with denial. Total disbelief, particularly if the event has been a stillbirth during labour, may affect their ability to care for the mother and to communicate properly (Jolly 1987). At a time when they should be particularly caring, they may appear detached and unsupportive.

Anger

'Why me?' Rage, envy and resentment accompany anger at the injustice of the situation, anger which can be let loose in all directions, making it an extremely difficult emotion for the staff and family to deal with. The feeling may be expressed simultaneously by both partners and directed at a particular person. Quite often innocent people are the targets, and inappropriate and unjust as this may seem there is very little one can do to avoid it. Underpinning all emotions will be the overbearing feeling of sadness. The sadness is hard to bear because there is nothing one can do to escape it; accepting it is not easy and the frustration leads to violent emotional outbursts (Kohner and Henley 1991; Mander 1994).

Anger may be intensified by the feeling of losing control in the medical setting – the absence of choice or a full understanding of what is happening (Jolly 1987). Once out in the open the anger can dissipate more quickly and will be less directed towards inappropriate people (Kennedy and Charles 1991). Other targets include family members or the partner, or turning the anger inwards. The danger with directing feelings inwardly is that they can present as depression, guilt or low self-esteem, which in turn may lead to suicidal thoughts (Worden 1992). For the woman, a decrease in hormonal levels associated with the ending of the pregnancy may significantly affect the coping mechanism and result in mood swings (Friedman and Gradstein 1992).

Siblings and friends may find themselves under attack, especially if they have children. Neighbours may inadvertently say the wrong thing and cause further upset and distress; angry words may be exchanged and lead to long-term difficulties. Returning to work may add increased stress; colleagues may have been unaware of the pregnancy and fail to offer expected support and sympathy. The expectation may be irrational, yet still cause conflict.

An apparently safe option would be to direct the anger towards the dead baby as an opportunity to express feelings of guilt and outrage without recriminations – did the baby do this on purpose? The pregnancy may have involved considerable time, effort and expenditure on the part of the parents, and this is how they have been repaid! Yet the memory of this pregnancy may haunt the couple and they must be encouraged to deal with it rather than always with the anger. Fear of future pregnancies will not be reduced if the baby is considered to have some control over the outcome.

Bargaining

> *The bargaining is really an attempt to postpone ...*
> (Kubler-Ross 1992)

Kubler-Ross identified the stage of bargaining in her work with the dying. She discovered that, by using various tools, terminally ill patients or their relatives would 'bargain' for a longer remission or, more often, life itself. The focal point for the transaction is whoever is deemed to be in control – God, doctors or the dying person themselves. The pregnant woman who is waiting for results of an amniocentesis may find herself making promises to God about her behaviour; for example 'I will attend church every week if the baby is OK'. Bargaining is not restricted to the immediate family who are involved, it can extend to anyone who knows the individual. Bargaining is a powerful tool in terms of hope. It is only when the time limit has expired that hope fades and is replaced by resentment. For example, the amniocentesis reveals a chromosomal defect and the mother swears that she will never set foot inside a church again.

The area of fetal loss in relation to bargaining has not been studied. Prenatal diagnosis affords some opportunity while waiting for results, but, for the majority of parents there is very little time available to bargain with.

Depression

For the postnatal mother who gave birth to a live baby, the third-day coincidence of a reduction in hormone levels, breastmilk coming in and the tiredness following childbirth is often sufficient to cause a mild depression. To the bereaved mother who experiences each of these effects, the discovery that her body continues to behave as though the baby were alive may only add further insult, sufficient in some instances to lead to a breakdown.

Following the death of their baby the couple may experience feelings of excessive sadness or hopelessness. Depression often gives rise to physical symptoms which, in the woman, are understandable following the actual delivery. Partners may find themselves confused at the physical manifestation of their depression; previous unresolved losses may surface as the pain of this death is felt. For many couples the loss of their baby may be the first confrontation they have had with death. It is possible that they will start to question their own mortality. [Particularly young or immature couples may start to question their own mortality. Their ability to understand or appreciate the significance of death may be limited.] They may rely heavily on health professionals and family members for support and guidance.

Acceptance

> *It is not in human nature to accept the finality of death*
> *without leaving a door open for some hope.*
>
> (Kubler-Ross 1992)

The acceptance of the death of a baby is a difficult concept for everyone involved. There may never be adequate answers to why it occurred. In her work Kubler-Ross discovered that the couples who do best are those who are encouraged to express their rage, to cry, to talk about their fears and fantasies. A sympathetic listener is important to this process.

Twenty years ago the management of stillborn babies focused on removing the evidence and forgetting the whole event. Heightened awareness of the need to grieve has enabled many women to come to terms with their loss and to reflect on the positive effects (Mooney 1985). A delay between the discovery of the death and the delivery may have allowed the couple to start working through some of the grieving process. This is not to suggest that preparation time means that the news is any less devastating, but these couples may reach a stage of acceptance sooner than others.

The fact also remains that some people never reach a true acceptance of the facts. They constantly strive to find out why the loss occurred, often trying to apportion blame which is unsubstantiated. An inability to accept the situation may preclude the person from moving on and continuing with their own life; relationships with others break down and isolation is increased.

THE MOURNERS

The mourning process is a convoluted one within which each person works at their own pace and may not be hurried. Acceptance of the needs of others is important when we are considering grieving: the partner, siblings, grandparents and relatives must all be allowed space to deal with the event in their own way.

The Partner

The partner may be male or female. Response to the death of 'their' baby will not depend on their biological input into the conception of the pregnancy. He or she may feel that it is his/her role to be strong and supportive until the delivery is complete; in most cases the partner is the main support for the client (Lewis 1994). Following this the partner may not be able to start their own grieving process and find that they have developed an inability to cope with their own emotions. The effect which this response can have on the relationship can be devastating. Rather than supporting each other through this traumatic period the couple may grow apart.

Focus and attention is aimed at the mother – she is the one who has to undergo the physical experience. Fear for her well-being may cause her partner greater distress, and associated with this may by a feeling of guilt. If the partner is a man, it may be guilt at his inability to go through the labour himself, guilt for the pain which the woman is suffering in a pregnancy which he feels responsible for. In times of stress the body reacts by a 'fight or flight' mechanism: unable to fight the actual event over which he or she has no control, the partner may escape from the scene. The ability to do this may heighten the guilt (Friedman and Gradstein 1992).

The duration of the pregnancy may determine the partner's response. If the pregnancy is well established, he or she is likely to have seen the ultrasound images of the baby, and this will make the pregnancy more of a reality. For the woman undergoing the pregnancy, her links with the baby evolve as she feels movements or notes the various body changes which occur in early pregnancy. Another important consideration for the partner is the degree to which the pregnancy was wanted in the first place; the response to the loss may be a direct reaction to the desire to be a father. In an all-female relationship the difficulties of conception and social acceptance of the child will have been an important preconceptual consideration. An unwanted pregnancy may result in a strong sense of loss and bereavement, but may also leave a feeling of relief behind. For a couple who have undergone extensive fertility treatment to achieve a pregnancy, the pregnancy may have more emphasis and the loss may involve more than this baby; it may include their dreams of ever having a child.

Suppression of emotions by the partner may manifest as problems later. Having kept a lid on their feelings until the initial 'crisis' has passed for the mother, the partner may find it difficult to let go and grieve. The amount of time which the client spends grieving may seem prolonged and it may be difficult to appreciate her needs. There may be an element of blame which each partner is secretly attaching to the other. Much will depend on the existing relationship before this tragedy occurred. Human nature is unpredictable; strong partnerships may flounder when confronted by a stillbirth, while less established relationships may be strengthened by the needs of the other.

The task of spreading the news to the rest of the family is usually undertaken by the partner (Lewis 1994). The difficulties involved in this are numerous and there is no easy approach to telling people bad news. The only positive aspect of informing friends and relatives is the support which is forthcoming. But even this is not guaranteed and may be directed towards the mother. Questions about how she is coping, followed by expressions of admiration, may leave the partner isolated and alone. This may be particularly so for the male partner, the presumption that he will cope because he is a man still being a powerful one (O'Dowd 1993). The death of a baby is likely to have the same devastating effect on a man as on a women, but the social acknowledgement and opportunity for expression is usually absent. While sympathetic friends offer the mother tissues and encourage her to express her grief, 'permission' for the father to weep for his loss may only come from his partner. Failing that he cries in secret, at night or in solitude. Work provides a comfort but also a barrier to the expression of grief (Knowles 1994; Mander 1994).

The Children

The temptation to protect children from the truth about death can be very strong, but to do so may suppress the child's grief and this may not become apparent until later in life (Stewart and Dent 1994). The decision when and how to inform siblings of the loss depends on the ages and abilities of those children. Parents should be encouraged to remember that children are very intuitive and can usually guess when something is wrong; it can be very confusing for them to be protected from bad news.

Worth bearing in mind is the fact that children view death in a more direct way than adults; to them the event is more straightforward and acceptable (Jolly 1987). Other than an inability to understand the reasons behind it there are very few grey areas to a child's attitude; also, they do not necessarily associate death with suffering as most adults do.

The terminology used to describe death to children must take account of their level of interpretation. To say that the baby is 'sleeping' rather than dead may confuse them when they note the amount of distress caused by this. In turn they may become frightened of falling asleep. 'Gone to heaven' is a common expression which may mean very little, especially to a child who has no concept of distances. However, using words like 'dead' may be very difficult for the mother and she may seek solace in the softer words. Staff cannot expect to influence the way parents deal with siblings, they can only provide a sounding board or offer helpful suggestions.

Children can also experience feelings of guilt, especially older children who may have resented the news of the pregnancy in the first place (Wathen 1990). If they have no explanation of the events, they may connect the death with their wishes and consider themselves responsible. Parents may have to overcome their own distress and discuss the death in a realistic manner with the siblings. For the child, seeing his parents in sorrow may be very upsetting but they are too wise to be unaware of a change in behaviour (Kohner and Henley 1991). Worden recommends the dispelling of 'magical and erroneous thinking regarding death' (Worden 1992).

The crucial aspect of bereavement is one which may affect their future development and ability to deal with relationships. Involving children in the period following delivery is still relatively uncommon. Eyebrows are raised by well-meaning staff at the suggestion that a child may see or hold his dead brother or sister. Projecting adult views onto children can prevent them from developing special memories of the baby. They may have been very involved in the growing pregnancy and want to know about the baby, to hold and have their photograph taken with her or him. Our attitude to encouraging parents to view the dead baby is based on helping them to ultimately accept the death. As Stewart reminds us, 'children have rights the same as adults' and offering the choice after gentle preparation can allow the child to make a decision which he can cope with (Stewart and Dent 1994).

The Grandparents

Grandchildren are fun, they provide all the enjoyment of having children without the responsibility. If both sets of grandparents are alive, there is the potential for the pregnancy to bring joy to four people; in today's society of divorce and remarriage this may extend even further. Regardless of how many grandchildren are already in the family, grandparents usually manage to stretch their love and affection around. Grandparents may not be old, they may still be of childbearing age themselves, and the support offered to the parents of the baby may be financial as well as emotional (Mander 1994).

The level of involvement in the pregnancy depends on the relationship with the mother-to-be. The grandmother is usually more closely linked to the antenatal period, having experienced the process herself. Grandfathers may adopt a more traditional male role in awaiting the time when the baby is in the cot to become involved. Yet the devastation wrought by the death of this baby can be overwhelming. It may be that they are unable to be physically close to the mother, in another country, or restricted by illness from travelling; any number of reasons may mean the news is relayed by telephone or letter. Sharing details of the loss may be difficult for the couple who are trying to come to accept the finality of it themselves. The family may be left bewildered, with many unanswered questions and nowhere to turn for help.

If the death is the result of a therapeutic termination of pregnancy, the grandparents may not be aware of all the facts. For people undergoing prenatal screening and diagnosis of abnormality, the language used and the interpretation of results may be too confusing to repeat. They may be too painful to discuss or considered too private. The couple may be concerned that their decision to terminate the pregnancy would be disapproved of by an older person. In any of these situations nurses or midwives may find themselves on the receiving end of questions from anxious grandparents. Gently guiding them towards the mother and supporting the mother's choice of communication is part of the care which can be extended to the grandparents.

The death of a baby is not a new phenomenon and grandparents may relive a personal experience from their past. Knowledge of an early loss may have been kept secret from the 'children'. It is very possible that the older couple did not have the opportunity to fully grieve for their loss. In silence, in private and alone they may have mourned for their dead child (Knowles 1994). The newly bereaved mother may be surprised to learn of her own mother's loss and gain comfort from a shared grief. The number of women (and men) who attend a Service of Remembrance in honour of their child who died twenty or thirty years previously is evidence that we are adopting the right approach in encouraging real mourning for a dead baby.

COUNSELLING

Where can these families turn for assistance? Professionally trained bereavement counsellors are available, but often it is a question of how to access the service. Self-help groups for bereaved parents such as the Stillbirth and Neonatal Death Society (SANDS) are evident in most areas of the country. The Miscarriage Association and Support After Termination for Abnormality (SATFA) are some of the agencies which have become established in the last ten years.

What about the immediate postnatal period? For the parents on the ward who have just delivered their much-wanted baby, the son or daughter who is about to be transferred to the mortuary rather than the nursery? For these parents it may be too early to deal with professional counsellors, the pain is too raw and recent. First they have to come to terms with the last twenty-four hours.

But they may still want to talk about the event. The option to talk to a professionally trained counsellor should be a standard in perinatal loss management and included in the purchasing of maternity services. Recognition of the need for professional counselling is becoming much more acceptable. Increasing numbers of nurses, doctors and midwives are enrolling for courses in basic counselling skills. At some time the very nature of nursing involves some form of counselling. Physically caring for people places the health professional in a position of vulnerability; it is a short step from this to emotional exposure. The client may choose to confide her problems to the most junior member of the team. Alternatively, the carer may consider that there is a problem to be addressed although the client is not ready to discuss it. Tschudin advises caution in that 'you cannot "counsel" someone; you can only help them to ask for counselling' (Tschudin 1991). The ability to counsel should not be regarded as a unique talent bestowed on a few, select individuals, nor should it be considered a 'mystique or special charisma' (Tschudin 1991). What is required of a non-professional counsellor are personal qualities which include flexibility, warmth, acceptance of others, open-mindedness, empathy, self-awareness, genuineness and respect for others (Kohner and Henley 1991; Tschudin 1991).

Counselling within a hospital is often undertaken in a crisis situation, in pain and at the height of the issue. As Tschudin points out it is difficult to know when caring stops and counselling starts. Nurses, midwives and doctors provide clients with direct physical care, they offer advice and guidance and they teach. Each is a caring or helping role. It is only when creating an environment which allows individuals to develop and meet their own needs that the health worker takes on a counselling role (Nurse 1978). Nurses are accustomed to problem solving and have to adapt to a problem-management position (Tschudin 1991).

Counselling requires courage and self-confidence. The nurse, midwife or doctor has to be comfortable with who they are. Trained or not, it is difficult for a counsellor to be totally objective and rational. To do so is to deny one's own feelings, ideas and perceptions (Munro et al 1990). Conflict of values is not a barrier to counselling, provided that the health professional is honest about his or her own beliefs and recognises the importance of not imposing them on others. The purpose of counselling is to increase the reality of the loss, not to judge. Differences in race, gender and culture are significant and should not be overlooked. The need to be aware of the ethnically sensitive and appropriate care of those suffering a perinatal loss is highlighted by the higher mortality rates in the non-white populations (Stewart and Dent

1994). Considerations of how various cultures grieve and support each other through the process is important.

The potential risk is that midwives, nurses and doctors who have not undergone any formal training will avoid any kind of counselling. The emphasis in maternity care today focuses heavily on the continuity of carer (Expert Maternity Group 1993). Midwives are encouraged to manage individual caseloads and accept the role of lead provider of care if that is the woman's choice. Care is transferred to a doctor if an abnormality is suspected or diagnosed, but the same midwife continues to provide the midwifery aspects. The more traditional system of maternity care tended to reflect greater continuity in the community setting; when a deviation from the norm was identified the woman would often be 'lost' to the hospital midwives and fragmentation of care would occur. The days of meeting thirty professionals during a single antenatal course are not completely gone, but much work to improve continuity and increase choice and control in childbirth is visible nationally.

The concept of a Named Midwife reaches some way to improving the care for women who are ultimately bereaved. Each health professional involved in providing the care has a greater opportunity to get to know the individual client and her particular needs. For midwives, managing their own women from booking the package will include the provision of care during labour. If a woman is admitted with an intrauterine death, the Named Midwife will attempt to be present for the delivery. In the case of a therapeutic termination of pregnancy, good practice would be to include the known midwife in planning the date for induction and aiming for him or her to provide care.

Advantages to the system of care include the relationship which the midwife has built up with the mother and possibly her partner from the beginning of the pregnancy. She will appreciate the significance of this baby to this particular couple. They will feel more confident to discuss the outcome with a familiar person, especially if they have 'unusual' requests, such as the desire to bury the baby in their garden. Knowing the couple enables the midwife to deal with situations in a more comfortable way than if she has just met them on the delivery suite.

A disadvantage of the continuity of carer may be that the midwife becomes the focus for blame. Being able to refuse the care of a particularly midwife is also to make an informed choice on the woman's part. For the midwifery manager understanding why the woman has declined an individual is important. The woman may choose not to disclose her reasons, in which case nothing much can be achieved other than to respect her wishes and replace the midwife. If the woman is prepared to talk about her concerns, then the midwifery manager should use the information constructively. A simple clash of personalities may be to blame and the situation may be an isolated incident. However, if there is something of greater concern, then the appropriate management action or the advice of a Supervisor of Midwives may be sought. All matters should be investigated thoroughly as with any suggestion of malpractice or negligence within the associated nursing, midwifery or medical professions.

RECOMMENDATIONS FOR GOOD PRACTICE

It is unrealistic to suggest that a single person can provide total continuity of care to a woman. Midwives and nurses will continue to look after women they have never met before the point of delivery; ultrasonographers will diagnose intrauterine deaths on strangers, and doctors will request postmortem consent from shocked clients who were expecting a birth certificate. What do they do if the woman breaks down and cries in front of them? How do they react if she decides that she wants to talk about her lost dreams when they need to get blood samples to the laboratory? What about the other women in labour?

It is rare for professionals to be able to devote their whole time to this one client. When labour is established, a midwife will be allocated to provide care for the client, but the focus is then on getting through the labour and it is rarely the time when she wants to talk and be 'counselled'. Regardless of how busy they are, it is important for the doctor or midwife to stop and acknowledge what the woman is saying. Trust is built up as faces become familiar.

Timing in these situations is never perfect; the changing face of nursing, midwifery and medical practice means that more acute care is delivered, there is a faster turnover of clients and less time to sit and talk. For the woman, awareness of the busy ward situation may prevent her from talking or leave her feeling guilty for taking up 'precious' time. In the present climate of purchaser/provider split between health authorities and hospital trusts, it is important that service specifications agreed by both parties recognise the need to provide trained counsellors to meet the needs of bereaved couples.

Recommendations for good counselling techniques are available in most textbooks on the subject. For the amateur counsellor, many of the 'rules' apply. Here the midwife, nurse or doctor is referred to as the 'counsellor'.

The counsellor should observe the following points.

- Acknowledge that the client is trying to talk about her feelings and grief.
- If it is inconvenient, explain why it is not possible to sit down and talk at this moment. Make a definite time to return, and keep the appointment.
- Allow space, in both personal and physical terms. Invasion of personal space is uncomfortable and to be avoided. Ensure that there are sufficient chairs in the room and try not to sit on the bed.
- Avoid standing over the client as this conveys a sense of impatience and does not provide a conducive setting for counselling.
- Inform colleagues of your whereabouts in order to avoid unnecessary interruptions. Bleeps and telephone enquiries should be handled by colleagues except in an emergency.
- The client should be advised of the amount of time which is available. The counsellor should avoid clock-watching as this may relay the wrong signals.

AIMS

The client may be numb and in a state of shock for some time following the delivery, yet express a desire to talk about the event. On reliving the experience many times the story changes, details are dropped or emerge, and it becomes more part of the person. In these circumstances what can the chosen counsellor hope to achieve?

- Relive the recent event of the labour and delivery.
- Provide an environment in which the bereaved parents can begin to acknowledge the reality of the loss.
- Deal with the expressed and latent effects of the death.
- Say an appropriate goodbye.

This is most likely to be achieved by the counsellor displaying genuineness, acceptance and empathetic understanding.

ASPECTS OF COUNSELLING

Many aspects of counselling are performed automatically and without thought. For some unskilled counsellors, however, concern may be expressed regarding the 'correct' approach if they suddenly get caught up with the emotion and start to cry.

Consideration is given here to the aspects of counselling which may be frightening and confusing if they occur.

Silence

Silence scares people within normal conversation. In a counselling situation with an untrained counsellor it can be embarrassing and frightening. The counsellor needs to accept the strength and power of silence (Kennedy and Charles 1991; Tschudin 1991), to use the silence effectively and have confidence in it, if possible allowing the woman to break it. It may be that the woman or her partner have stopped at a particular point and require some prompting to move on. Recognising that they need time to absorb and reflect in silence, the counsellor avoids rushing them forward.

Tears

Crying in front of a relative stranger is not a comfortable experience for most people. Tears indicate despair and this can be difficult to witness. But crying can be vital to the grieving process and should not be discouraged; the family may require encouragement to understand this concept. Time limits are often applied to the length of crying the bereaved is supposed to do. 'She's cried enough' or 'I don't know where all the tears came from' are common enough statements. The counsellor will encourage the woman to apply her own limitations to personal grief. The couple who have just lost their baby have a lot to cry about.

What of the health professional who breaks down? Is this wrong or unprofessional? The answer lies in the relationship which he or she has with the woman. To many couples, the knowledge that their loss has affected the staff may help them. It may acknowledge the tragedy and place a significance on it enabling them to realise that this is not an everyday event and that each situation is personal and individual. Sometimes an expression of feeling on the part of the professional can be extremely appropriate (Kennedy and Charles 1991). So tears are acceptable, provided that the bereaved couple do not feel that they must support the doctor or midwife.

Listening

The art of listening is important to all counselling (Jolly 1987; Kennedy and Charles 1991; Tschudin 1991). The listener needs to be at the same height as the speaker – towering above her can be intimidating, especially if she is in a bed. Placing a chair in the correct position is an important detail to consider when talking to someone who is upset. It is then necessary for the counsellor to listen attentively. Body language gives clues about the importance with which the message is being received. The counsellor should be facing the woman and look her in the eye when she speaks. Fidgeting is forbidden and posture should be upright. When listening attentively, minimum gestures of appreciation should be used – a nod or shake of the head, single words, gentle noises. Tschudin recommends similar behaviour to that which is employed when watching television (Tschudin 1991). Active listening involves a great deal of silence on the counsellor's part. The art of listening uses all senses in order to obtain the total message:

> *listen with the ears to the words spoken ... with the mind to the underlying message ... with the eyes to the body language.*
> (Tschudin 1991)

Touch

To touch another individual is to invade their personal space. It suggests familiarity with the person and may have cultural significance in some societies. The physical nature of childbirth makes a tactile approach less threatening and more comforting. It is easier for the midwife who has delivered the baby to put her arm around the mother or her partner when they cry. Touching a bereaved mother may speak volumes more than a thousand words; in a simple embrace the midwife can express concern and caring for the individual; holding her hand can offer lasting sympathy and indicates that she is not alone.

Information Gathering

Asking the right questions in order to gain information can be difficult. Although the circumstances of the loss will be well known to the counsellor, there may be a particular aspect which is causing greater concern. Discovering what this is requires patience and understanding. The woman may not know what the problem is; perhaps she is complaining of physical symptoms which will enable her to stay in hospital and avoid returning home to an empty cot. If the medical staff are unable to find a problem they must gently probe deeper in order to establish the real worry. Open-ended questions invite her to continue talking by suggesting that she gives more detail. Closed questions require only yes or no responses and can tend to resemble an interrogation, shutting off a conversation and implicitly suggesting that she answer only what is asked of her (Tschudin 1991). Open questions are useful for discovering opinions and explanations from the couple; they offer free information to be followed up and keep the interview going. Munro et al highlight that it is important that open questions are not thought of as 'good' counselling skills while closed questions are considered 'bad'. Both can be effective when used properly.

Accepting

To be non-judgemental and encourage the client to talk freely is important: accepting what is said without criticism, enabling the freedom of speech which may be irrational and contradicted later. Confidence in the listener allows this process to occur and continuity with the carer is an important factor in this.

THE NEXT STEP

Following the intense period around the time of birth, the woman has to return to her own environment. For many women this is a difficult step. Some are keen to leave hospital as quickly as possible, a place associated with the death of their baby, and they may find it too traumatic to return to the same hospital in the future. For others the hospital provides a safe haven, somewhere for them to hide and be cared for, allowing midwifery, nursing and medical staff to make decisions for them. They do not have to worry about the shopping or paying bills, nor do they have to face the preparations which were made for the baby's safe arrival.

The transition back into the community is eased by the presence of a familiar midwife, hopefully someone who was very involved and aware of the situation. If the woman has not received continuity with the visiting midwife (perhaps she had a termination of pregnancy in another hospital far from home), communication between the discharging hospital and community staff must be of a high standard and ensure that details are passed on. Regardless of the gestation reached, a visit may be offered from a midwife. The midwife will try to be aware of the needs of this individual and how to facilitate those needs; she will be in a position to witness how the woman resumes her own life and to assist with some of the difficulties. As a person to whom the woman can turn and talk without fear of causing upset, the General Practitioner can also fulfil this role and it is equally important that he or she is aware of the outcome of the pregnancy.

Funeral arrangements may need to be made and this can give some focus to the immediate postnatal period. Worden considers a funeral to be an important 'adjunct in aiding and abetting the healthy resolution of grief' (Worden 1992). Advice on how to arrange a funeral may be sought from the midwife or doctor, who will require knowledge about who to contact to arrange this as highlighted in Chapter 8 on Funeral Arrangements.

Adjustment to a more normal routine will vary according to individual needs and the circumstances surrounding the perinatal loss. Days will pass which are relatively calm and with little distress, then an event may occur which brings home the truth, perhaps a neighbour innocently asking about the outcome of the pregnancy. Embarrassment and distress about how to handle these situations are not easy to overcome; preparing the couple in advance may help. Advice regarding whom to inform and how to go about that process may ease some of the difficulties in the months ahead. Returning to work is another milestone, again depending on the gestation and how aware colleagues were of the pregnancy.

Other Agencies

The Stillbirth and Neonatal Death Society (SANDS), Support After Termination for Abnormality (SATFA), The Miscarriage Association, National Childbirth Trust (NCT), Relate (Marriage Guidance Council) and the British Association for Counselling are all agencies which help people come to terms with bereavement. Many are self-referral and information may be given to the couple by the hospital or primary care team.

The classic situation involves the midwife giving the contact telephone number for the local SANDS befriender to the mother; the midwife does not 'refer' the woman herself, rather she explains the nature of the work undertaken by SANDS. The woman is discharged and receives support from her partner, family and friends, time passes, and life begins to resume a more normal pattern; she has started working again, perhaps becoming absorbed in her other children or outside interests. One day, out of the blue and totally unexpectedly, she is overwhelmed by grief for the loss she has experienced. It may be difficult to find a sympathetic ear; glances tell her that she is expected to be over this by now. To whom can she turn? Then she remembers the telephone number in her purse and makes the call herself. From this point she is in contact with at least one person who has shared her experience, perhaps in very different circumstances but someone who understands the pain and the fear associated with its return. The next step depends on her; she may be comfortable with a person to whom she can turn via the telephone, or as a couple they may attend support sessions at the house of another bereaved couple.

For some women this may not be sufficient or there may not be a local SANDS group. She may turn instead to her GP, who may make the professional decision that help is required in the form of a trained counsellor. Referral is then made to an appropriate source.

COMPLETION OF THE MOURNING PROCESS

The completion of the period of mourning depends solely on the individual concerned. Unreal expectations can result in complications of grieving; if an individual believes that she will have recovered from this loss in four weeks, she will have problems coping with the fact that she still feels an acute loss months later. The twelve-month cycle is considered to be more realistic, although Worden suggests two years (Worden 1992). Twelve months allows the passage of the same seasons through which the pregnancy occurred, it covers the delivery period and also the expected date of delivery. Instead of 'This time last year I was pregnant', it puts a whole year between the past and the present. The expected date of confinement may be very difficult for the couple to deal with, especially if it is some months from the death. For some women it is a milestone of which they are ever conscious and afraid of how they will deal with it. Partners may take time off work and the day may include visiting the graveside or looking through the mementoes such as the footprints and photographs (Mallinson 1989). For a woman who has a surviving baby, the date of birth may be as significant as the date of death. These parents have to adapt to sharing a joyful reminder of life with the grief of a death.

Gradual acceptance of the loss will develop. It is important for the couple to accept that this particular baby is irreplaceable. Nothing will ever completely fill the gap which has been caused by this death; no future baby will ever be a substitute for the one who has died.

FUTURE PLANS

Contraception

Contraceptive advice ought to be covered while the woman is still in hospital. She may not be very receptive at the time, but it is important that the next pregnancy is planned rather than an 'accident'. If a subsequent pregnancy occurs before the grieving process has been worked through, then a holding relationship may be established for the gestation period (Lewis 1994). With the delivery of the baby there may be a severe grief reaction to the previous loss.

CONCLUSION

The term 'counsellor' may be frightening to the midwife, doctor or nurse, who may feel unsuited to the role. In reflecting on the role which they do fulfil, health professionals may be surprised to discover that they are meeting the needs of clients in a counselling capacity on a daily basis. The difference is applying the formal title to the role. Fear of saying or doing the 'wrong thing' may prevent staff from listening or talking to the woman and her partner. Confidence is gained from experience, the ability to discuss the issues and situations with colleagues and peers, and seeking advice from a variety of resources; knowing when to refer to others and when a listener is all that is required.

REFERENCES

Department of Health (1994) *Report on the Confidential Enquiry into Maternal Deaths in the UK 1988–90.* London, HMSO.

Expert Maternity Group (1993) *Changing Childbirth*, Part 1. London, HMSO.

Friedman R & Gradstein B (1992) *Surviving Pregnancy Loss.* London, Little Brown.

Jolly J (1987) *Missed Beginnings: Death Before Life Has Been Established.* Lisa Sainsbury Foundation Series.

Kennedy E & Charles SC (1991) *On Becoming a Counsellor: A Basic Guide for Non-professional Counsellors.* Dublin, Gill & Macmillan.

Knowles S (1994) A passage through grief: the Western Australia Rural Pregnancy Loss Team. *British Medical Journal* **309**: 1705–1708.

Kohn I & Moffitt P-L (1994) When an unborn or newborn baby dies. In *Pregnancy Loss*, pp 3–21. London, Hodder & Stoughton.

Kohner N & Henley A (1991) The experience of late miscarriage, stillbirth and neonatal death. In *When a Baby Dies*. London, Pandora Press.

Kubler-Ross E (1992) *On Death and Dying*. London, Routledge.

Lewis H (1994) Coping with stillbirth. *New Society* 8 Apr.: 64.

Mallinson G (1989) When a baby dies. *Nursing Times* **85**: 31–34.

Mander R (1994) Grieving, mourning, loving and losing. In *Loss and Bereavement in Childbearing*, pp 1–17. Oxford, Blackwell Scientific Publications.

COUNSELLING – Future Plans

Mooney B (1985) The spirit cannot die. *The Listener* 14 Nov.: 29.

Munro A, Manthei B & Small J (1990) *Counselling: The Skills of Problem Solving*. London, Routledge.

Nurse G (1978) What is counselling? *Midwife, Health Visitor and Community Nurse* 14: 352–355.

O'Dowd T (1993) The needs of fathers. *British Medical Journal* **306**: 1484–1485.

Parkes CM (1970) The first year of bereavement: A longitudinal study of the reaction of London widows to deaths of husbands. *Psychiatry* **33**: 444–467.

Stewart A & Dent A (1994) Understanding loss and bereavement. In (A Stewart & A Dent, eds) *At A Loss* pp 1–12. London, Baillière Tindall.

Theut S, Henderson F, Zaslow M, Cain R, Rabinovich B & Morihisa J (1989) Perinatal loss and perinatal bereavement. *Journal of Psychiatry* **146**: 635–639.

Tschudin V (1991) *Counselling Skills for Nurses*. London, Baillière Tindall.

Wathen NC (1990) Perinatal bereavement. *British Journal of Obstetrics and Gynaecology* **97**: 759–761.

Worden JW (1992) Grieving special types of loss. In *Grief Counselling and Grief Therapy*. London, Tavistock Publications.

Chapter Three

Spontaneous Abortion

Spontaneous abortion, commonly known as a 'miscarriage', is a term used to describe the expulsion of the products of conception before the fetus has reached the 24-week age of viability. Fifteen per cent of all clinically recognised pregnancies are complicated by spontaneous abortion. The classical presentation is vaginal bleeding, with or without abdominal cramps. The bleeding may be due to a variety of causes ranging from implantation of the ovum to an ectopic pregnancy or a warning sign of an impending miscarriage. A threatened abortion or miscarriage is not an uncommon event. There are an estimated 700,000 threatened abortions in England and Wales each year; around 50–70% of these pregnancies progress normally with no increased risk of abnormality (Allan 1993).

A percentage of spontaneous abortions (estimated to be 25%) remain undetermined in their aetiology, mostly because of the lack of ability to investigate the individual cases (Edmunds 1992). Of those which are investigated, a variety of causes are identified. Categories include genetic factors, developmental problems, placental problems and infection. The process of abortion is often considered to be the route by which natural selection operates in humans.

INEVITABLE ABORTION

In the case of an inevitable abortion the contents of the uterus are not completely expelled and the bleeding can continue, accompanied by severe stomach cramps. The pain is due to cervical dilatation which is secondary to uterine contractions resulting from prostaglandin release as the placenta and membranes separate from the uterine site. Blood loss may be considerable and the woman may present with shock; this may be secondary to the haemorrhage or due to products of conception being held in the cervix, leading to a sympathetic stimulation. Gentle vaginal examination will reveal the latter, the removal of which will relieve the symptoms of shock (Edmunds 1992). Admission to hospital is usually required and the evacuation of the uterine contents may be performed under general anaesthetic.

In the case of a complete abortion, the conceptus is totally expelled from the uterus and the signs of pregnancy diminish. A complete abortion is more common after 16 weeks but the potential for a secondary haemorrhage or an infection should not be overlooked. Prior to discharge from hospital the woman should be informed of the possible signs of infection such as feeling hot and having a temperature, bleeding or any persistent discomfort, and advised to contact her doctor with any queries. The hospital is responsible for ensuring that the GP receives a discharge summary of the woman's history and treatment (Allan 1993).

MISSED ABORTION

A missed abortion may be referred to as a blighted ovum or a carneous mole. In this event there is failure of embryonic growth in spite of placental viability, or a viable fetus dies. Fetal demise occurs before eight weeks, although the uterus does not expel the products. A brown vaginal discharge may be present, caused by increasingly non-viable placental tissue (Edmunds 1992). The discharge may be considered a threatened miscarriage, but this may settle and give false reassurance that the pregnancy is progressing normally. Concern will be expressed when the woman reports a disappearance of the signs of pregnancy. The diagnosis may be confirmed by ultrasound scan. The expulsion of the mole will occur spontaneously, but this may take several weeks so the woman is usually offered an evacuation of the uterus under general anaesthetic.

Prescribing bedrest for the woman with a threatened miscarriage is unlikely to make any difference to the outcome; the woman may feel that she is doing something positive to save the pregnancy but may also feel responsible for contributing to the loss if she has not rested previously. The same is true of advice to refrain from sexual intercourse. There are no studies available to suggest that this management has any bearing on the outcome of the pregnancy (Edmunds 1992).

If the abortion does occur unexpectedly at home, the woman is likely to be shocked. If there has been an opportunity to prepare the woman for the prospective loss of the pregnancy, staff will need to discuss the practical aspects of this. If the woman experiences severe stomach cramps, she may miscarry on the lavatory, a distressing event for her to come to terms with. It is not unusual for women to be admitted as an emergency case and to bring the result of their miscarriage to hospital with them. Knowing what to do with recognisable products of conception can be very difficult. Staff in the Accident & Emergency Department and the gynaecology ward need to handle the situation with great sensitivity, particularly as they are unlikely to be in full possession of the facts on immediate admission and so have no idea of how precious this pregnancy is to the individual.

Edmunds (1992) outlines some key points in the case of spontaneous abortion:

- The process of abortion is the major route by which natural selection operates in humans, with 50% of all clinically recognised first trimester losses being chromosomally abnormal.
- Abnormal placentation may be important in the aetiology of chromosomally normal spontaneous abortions: some may be amenable to treatment.
- Spontaneous abortion may result from isolated placental and fetal infections.
- The risk of spontaneous abortion in a clinically recognised pregnancy is around 15%.
- Women who suffer a threatened abortion are prone to late pregnancy complications and must be identified as a high-risk group.
- Psychological factors may adversely affect pregnancy outcome and therapy may improve reproductive performance.

EXPERIENCING SPONTANEOUS ABORTION

The presentation of a woman with a history of vaginal bleeding and abdominal pain in the early part of pregnancy is indicative of a threatened abortion. For the woman the situation may be very new and she will be confused and scared for the pregnancy and her own health. She may be unaware that she is even pregnant and be placed in a situation where she is grieving for a baby she did not realise she was carrying. The circumstances behind the pregnancy may be varied and include a poor obstetric history of recurrent miscarriage or a long period of infertility. For the nurse in the Accident and Emergency Department the additional support required may be a new area of care. Liaison with the gynaecology ward and the midwifery unit will help the staff to ensure that agreed standards are upheld.

Confirmation that the pregnancy has ended may be very upsetting for the couple and it is important that they have some privacy and time to ask questions. Unfortunately, in a busy casualty department this may be difficult. Deciding where to move the woman will depend on hospital policy. Normally she will be moved to a gynaecology ward if she is at less than 18 weeks gestation. The delivery suite is another option and the increase in day surgery units makes that another possibility if an evacuation of the uterus is required.

REFERENCES

Allan AN (1993) Management of vaginal bleeding in early pregnancy. *Update* May: 791–792.

Edmunds DK (1992) Spontaneous and recurrent abortion. In (R Shaw, P Souter & S Stanton, eds) *Gynaecology*, pp 205–218. Edinburgh, Churchill Livingstone.

Chapter Four

Therapeutic Termination of Pregnancy

Legal termination of pregnancy is available to women in the United Kingdom. There are five certified grounds for carrying out the procedure (Department of Health 1967):

- Continuation of the pregnancy would involve risk to the life of the pregnant woman greater than if the pregnancy were terminated.
- Termination is necessary to prevent grave permanent injury to the physical or mental health of the pregnant woman.
- The pregnancy has *not* exceeded its 24th week and the continuance of the pregnancy would involve risk, greater than if the pregnancy were terminated, of injury to the physical or mental health of the pregnant woman.
- The pregnancy has *not* exceeded its 24th week and the continuance of the pregnancy would involve risk, greater than if the pregnancy were terminated, of injury to the physical or mental health of any existing child(ren) of the family of the pregnant woman.
- There is a substantial risk that if the child were born it would suffer from such physical or mental abnormalities as to be seriously handicapped.

During the early months of the pregnancy a series of antenatal screening tests are offered to women. Routine antenatal serum screening commenced in the 1940s, and the discovery of the Rhesus factor in 1940 meant that babies at risk of iso-immunisation could be identified. Screening for rubella was started after the association between the virus and severe congenital abnormalities was recognised by an Australian obstetrician in 1941 (Tew 1995).

      Enkin et al (1990) argue that care during pregnancy should be effective, while *Changing Childbirth* places emphasis on empowering women to make informed choices about their maternity care (Department of Health 1967). Yet many do not understand the reason for the tests which they routinely undergo (Parry 1993a). If there is a lack of appreciation of the 'routine' tests of pregnancy, how easy is it to explain the more complex investigations which may be required? Why does this lack of understanding exist? *Changing Childbirth* goes on to say 'all women should have access to information about the services available in their locality' (Department of Health 1993).

There is a need for providers to supply information on all routine as well as specialised prenatal investigations. Feedback from consumers through a variety of questionnaires, comment cards, focus groups and Maternity Service Liaison Committees would benefit the provider by auditing the information given. It is not until one has experienced the system that omissions generally reveal themselves, therefore relying on the consumers to tell us would highlight areas to improve upon. The manner in which the information is published has to take account of the particular cultural and ethnic population served. Audio tapes may assist non-English-speaking, non-reading women. Purchasers are in a position to ensure that appropriate literature is available by including it in the service specification which is agreed with the provider prior to the contract being signed.

Antenatal care should ensure that the woman feels supported and fully informed throughout the pregnancy (Department of Health 1993). In her book *Safer Childbirth*, Tew (1995) argues that the technical advances made in the care of pregnant women have enabled obstetricians to know much more about the detection of abnormalities of pregnancy than the cure:

> *Unfortunately, ingenuity in inventing diagnostic techniques has far outstripped ingenuity in developing curative therapies; the new powers to diagnose have not yet been matched by new powers to cure.*

(Tew 1995)

ANTENATAL SCREENING TESTS

Throughout the course of a pregnancy a variety of screening tests are performed, some on a regular basis and a number according to individual need (Table 4.1). At the onset of pregnancy a gathering of information occurs to be used as a baseline for the antenatal course. For example, by assessing the haemoglobin level in early pregnancy the midwife can predict the possibility of the client having problems with anaemia later; this can be averted by good dietary and health advice and referral to a doctor for additional advice if necessary. Some tests are carried out at each antenatal visit; these include urinalysis, which checks for protein, glucose and ketones. If proteinuria is untreated, it can result in a urinary tract infection which could lead to a number of serious complications, including preterm labour. The detection of proteinuria at a routine analysis would indicate the need for further investigation, for which a midstream sample of urine would be required.

Of the routine screening tests, a number are performed on serum samples. It is important that a clear explanation is given prior to the taking of blood as the woman may misinterpret the intention. Screening is generally for rubella, syphilis, haemoglobin, antibody tests and hepatitis. In some areas hepatitis is not a routine test, and is only performed on 'high-risk' clients. Electrophoresis is particularly important for women at risk of sickle cell disease or thalassaemia. If the client tests positive to either of the latter, her partner should also be tested and they may then be referred for genetic screening. The midwife requires a clear understanding of the implications of these conditions to be able to offer choice to the woman.

Testing for the human immunodeficiency virus (HIV) is being conducted in some antenatal clinics. The arrangement generally consists of a trained counsellor who offers pre- and post-test counselling to the woman; the decision about whether to have the test rests with the individual client. If she chooses to do so, full confidentiality is maintained and she ought to decide who is given the information if she tests positive. A full paediatric support service should be in place for the care of the neonate. In addition, liaison with the physicians will become necessary if she develops symptoms during the pregnancy. If the woman chooses not to reveal her results, her decision must be respected. It has to be recognised that counsellors will be carrying this information and providing support: they also need support and should have access to a supervised session for themselves.

Attention to the local population must be given with regard to HIV. Where there is a particular ethnic group at risk of the virus, myths and suspicions may exist about the hospital care. One such myth is that the hospital tests the individual and arranges treatment and then the person dies; the society may interpret this as some evil on the part of the hospital to rid society of this 'menace'. As the rumour spreads, so patients show reluctance to be admitted; consequently their condition is much more severe and difficult to treat and the mortality rate increases, leading to greater suspicion. All of these aspects must be taken into account when one is considering the provision of the service to the local catchment area.

Table 4.1 Antenatal screening tests

Screening test	Gestation at which performed	Purpose of test	Routine or requested	Risk to fetus	Further investigations
Chorionic villus sampling	8–10 weeks	Karyotyping. Sex of the fetus. Diagnosing sickle cell disease or trait. Diagnosing thalassaemia	Requested	2–3%	Depends on findings
Cordocentesis	18 weeks	Identify haemoglobinopathies. Rapid karyotyping. Liver (fetal) biopsy	Requested	1%	Depends on findings
Human immunodeficiency virus (HIV)	Any gestation	To detect presence of virus in client	Requested	Nil	If test positive, then further investigation
Blood					
ABO group	Booking history	Knowledge of blood group for rapid cross match	Routine	Nil	Nil
Rhesus antibodies	Booking history	Detect antibodies – especially if mother is Rhesus negative	Routine	Nil	Antibodies present: repeat in third trimester. Cordocentesis if there are raised antibody levels
Serology	Booking history	Detect syphilis	Routine	Nil	Confirmatory tests
Haemoglobin estimation	Booking history	Detect anaemia	Routine	Nil	Repeat at regular intervals (varies but approximately 32 and 36 weeks). Further investigation required if anaemia is present
Haemoglobinopathies	Booking history	Detect sickle cell disease or trait. Detect thalassaemia major or minor	Requested for people of African, Asian or Mediterranean origin. Requested for partner if he is the above	Nil	Positive result, refer to genetic counselling
Rubella screening	Booking history	Detect non-immunity client	Routine	Nil	Rubella vaccine offered in postnatal period

Test	Timing	Purpose	Routine/requested	Risk	Notes
Hepatitis screening	Booking history	Detect surface antigen positive	Routine/requested	Nil	Nil
Urinalysis	Booking history/each antenatal visit	Detect proteinuria, glycosuria or ketones	Routine	Nil	Repeat at each antenatal visit. Midstream urine glucose tolerance test or/and fasting blood sugar. Further investigations depending on results
Blood pressure	Booking history/each antenatal visit	Detect hypertension	Routine	Nil	Depends on finding. Further investigation for pre-eclampsia or pregnancy induced hypertension
Ultrasound scan	16–18 weeks	Establish correct gestational age. Diagnose multiple pregnancy. Diagnose fetal abnormality. Localise the placenta	Routine	Nil	Depends on findings. Further ultrasound scan or screening tests may be indicated
Serum alphafetoprotein (αFP)	15–19 weeks	Detect neural tube defect in the fetus	Routine/requested	Nil	Ultrasound scan required before test to accurately date the pregnancy. Repeat αFP if positive. Anomaly scan if positive
Triple test (Barts test, Leeds test, serum screen)	10–13 weeks (up to 16 weeks)	Use of biochemical markers to indicate risk of Down's syndrome	Routine/requested	Nil	If markers are raised, then further investigation recommended – amniocentesis
Nuchal skin thickness	10–13 weeks	Measures the fetal nuchal fold to assess presence of Down's syndrome	Requested	Nil	Amniocentesis for karyotyping
Amniocentesis	16–18 weeks (as early as 10 weeks in some cases)	Chromosomal studies. Sex of the fetus. Rhesus incompatibility (to measure bilirubin)	Requested	1% due to spontaneous abortion or infection	Depends on findings

Recording of the woman's blood pressure is performed at each antenatal visit. Again the significance of the screening is to avoid complications associated with pre-eclampsia or pregnancy-induced hypertension. The management of essential hypertension must be carefully controlled during pregnancy, so it is necessary to identify the condition early if it has been undetected.

Weighing of clients is no longer routine in all antenatal clinics. It may be the woman's choice to know how much she is gaining but it has very little to do with the health of the pregnancy. Day-to-day fluctuations occur and this affects the weekly or longer pattern of assessment (Altman and Hytten 1993).

A cervical smear may be taken at the first booking visit. This will depend on the date of the last smear; alternatively, the smear may be left to the six-weeks postnatal check.

The tests referred to so far have been a combined screening process for maternal and fetal well-being. A mother with hypertension is likely to be unwell herself, but in addition her baby may suffer from diminished placental blood flow and impaired growth. A series of screening tests are available which focus directly on the fetus; some are offered as routine in most hospitals, others vary from place to place while a few are only available at specialist centres. Examples of the more commonly found screening tests are ultrasound scanning and biochemical screening (known as the Barts Test, the Leeds Test, or the Triple Test, each of which is considered in more detail below. Access to all tests should be possible for all pregnant women. Factors affecting the availability of tests include the availability of trained personnel, relevant experience and financial resources.

In some instances, such as a previously affected pregnancy or a family history of note, the couple may anticipate the need for specific screening. For others the request to carry out further tests may be an unexpected suggestion. Clear, concise communication is necessary regardless of whether the screening test is part of a routine investigation or for the specific detection of a fetal abnormality. In hospital people are surprisingly willing to allow their bodies to be prodded and to produce specimens without fully understanding the reasons. It is left to the professional to recognise the need to provide a more detailed explanation. The same is true of pregnant women who permit routine non-invasive testing to occur, often without knowing the significance. A lack of communication may be corrected later. For example, without understanding the significance of haemoglobin levels a woman allows the sample to be taken, and then receives a telephone call from the midwife advising her about iron supplements. Recognising her lack of appreciation, the midwife now has the opportunity to explain the investigation and the pregnancy continues, healthier for it.

Prenatal screening is undertaken in addition to the routine investigations of pregnancy. In order for the woman and her partner to make an informed choice, the midwife or doctor must have a comprehensive understanding of the additional tests available within their hospital or health authority. Certain tests are invasive in nature and the explanation must take this into account. It is those less-invasive tests which, on the surface, appear relatively harmless that often present the greatest dilemma. Universal acceptance of the ultrasound scan as a means of providing positive news of the pregnancy can lead to tremendous problems if an abnormality is discovered.

A study by Smith and Marteau (1995) looked at the information given to pregnant women when screening for fetal abnormality. In 215 antenatal consultations they found that very little information was routinely given to women about screening tests. If the information was given, the emphasis was on the practical aspects of the tests. Midwives were shown to be better than their obstetric colleagues at telling women what to expect and were more apt to describe the conditions being screened for. There was a tendency to spend time explaining particular investigations such as serum screening. The authors suggested that this may be because of greater knowledge about the specific investigation, or because the ultrasound scan was not perceived by the professional to merit the term 'invasive procedure'. In Nottingham an audit into serum screening for Down's syndrome revealed that women had a poor understanding of the reason for or the implications of the test (Newton and Walker 1994).

Screening for fetal abnormalities is usually undertaken for a particular reason. The list includes raised maternal age (generally considered to be 35 and above); a suspected abnormality found on a routine investigation; a family history of a congenital problem; or a previously affected pregnancy.

Raised Maternal Age

For a variety of reasons women are having babies later in their reproductive life, a fact which increases their likelihood of losing the pregnancy naturally or of having a baby with a chromosomal abnormality (Parry 1993a; Kohn and Moffitt 1994a). It is for the latter reason that women are referred to genetic counselling. The chance of a woman having a baby with Down's syndrome at the age of 25 is 1: 1376; at the age of 35 years the incidence has increased to 1: 424 and by 45 years is as high as 1: 31 (Wald 1984).

Suspected Abnormality on Routine Screening

The woman who has no family history, has never had an affected
child and who is not considered to be at risk may, nevertheless, be
referred for prenatal testing or counselling. The most likely reason
is that a routine investigation during the pregnancy has revealed a
potential problem; for example, the couple may be carriers of the
gene for sickle cell disease.

Family History of an Abnormality

In the ideal world, screening for inherited genetic disease should
be carried out before conception (Royal College of Physicians
1989). This does not always happen since the majority of couples
do not know they have a risk factor and so do not seek advice.
Fewer than 3% of pregnancies with a chromosomal abnormality
have no identifiable risk factors in the preconceptual period
(Nicolaides et al 1992).

The offending gene in a genetic abnormality may be
autosomal recessive or autosomal dominant. If both parents are
carriers of an autosomal recessive gene, then the child has a 1 in 4
chance of being affected and a 50% chance of becoming a carrier.
Haemoglobinopathies such as sickle-cell disease or thalassaemia
are examples of autosomal recessive diseases. Carriers of
haemoglobinopathies who choose a partner within their own
ethnic group have a 3–20% chance of forming a risk couple. The
rate of first-cousin marriages (consanguinity) among British
Pakistanis is 55% compared with 32% in Pakistan (OPCS 1986).
Sickle-cell disease and thalassaemia affect the population
originating from Africa, the Mediterranean, the Middle East and
parts of Asia.

In the case of an autosomally dominant gene the affected
parent is likely to be heterozygous, that is they have a normal gene
in addition to the abnormal one. The chance of the parent passing
on the affected gene is then 50%. The autosome will always
override the normal gene from the other parent and the baby will
be affected. An example of an autosomal dominant disease is
Huntington's chorea.

Some inherited genetic disorders are sex-linked, whereby
male children are affected and the females become carriers. The
most common example of this is haemophilia. Where the mother is
the carrier and the father is normal, their male children have a
50% chance of being affected by the disorder while the females
have a 50% chance of being carriers (Pembrey 1987; Royal College
of Physicians 1989; Parry 1993a).

Previously Affected Pregnancy

The offer of prenatal testing should be made to all couples with a previously affected pregnancy. The offer of prenatal testing should be available preconceptually. If the original relationship has ended and the couple have moved on to new partners, it is important that each has an understanding of the problem and is able to access help and advice in the future.

REFERRAL TO ADDITIONAL SCREENING

The need for additional screening having been identified, the woman should be referred as soon as possible. Considerable time may elapse before results are available. Owing to the complexity and level of expertise required to perform some of the additional screening tests and the fact that prenatal diagnosis is still a developing area, it may be necessary to refer the couple to a regional centre. For example, the opportunity to perform a cordocentesis may not occur very often in a small hospital. Lack of experience may affect the success of the sampling and therefore the results. The European trial on chorionic villus sampling (CVS) noted that '... safety of procedures such as CVS may be affected by the skill of the operator improving with experience' (MRC Working Party 1991).

Cost is also a factor when considering other tests. For example, a particular screening test for Down's syndrome (see under Biochemical Screening below) requires dye for analysis; the cost may prohibit the availability of the dye in all hospital laboratories and it may be more cost-effective to send the sample to another hospital. Sending the samples out for analysis should not inconvenience the couple. Specimens can be obtained by the midwife or the GP and the couple need not even know that the analysis is being conducted by another laboratory.

Genetic counselling is an inherent component of the process of prenatal diagnosis and is associated with the provision of a complete service. The first clinical genetics service was established in the United Kingdom in 1946; the aim was to gain greater understanding and knowledge of the nature of genetic disorders. In 1989 a report by the Royal College of Physicians defined the following objectives:

> To allow the widest possible range of informed choice to women and couples at risk of having children with an abnormality.

To provide reassurance and reduce the level of anxiety associated with reproduction.

To allow couples at risk to embark on having a family knowing that they may avoid the birth of seriously affected children through selective abortion.

To ensure optimal treatment of affected infants through early diagnosis.
(Royal College of Physicians, 1989)

The aim of genetic counselling is to provide couples with a non-directional approach to their individual pregnancy. For the woman and her partner to make an informed choice they must have as much information as possible. This includes the implications of various screening and invasive tests. It is not uncommon for pregnant women to know of screening tests, but Newton and Walker found that interpretation of biochemical screening tests was variable among lay women and misconceptions often exist. They suggest that:

a large-scale study of consumers' views ... would have been helpful in assessing consumers' needs and should provide a sound basis before the introduction of such a test.
(Newton and Walker 1994)

The couple should understand what each test is capable of looking for and the limitations of that test. Expecting an amniocentesis to provide information on actual physical handicaps is unrealistic and this should be explained beforehand. The diagnostic method of identifying babies with chromosomal disorders is amniocentesis or chorionic villus sampling; in either of these methods fetal cells are collected, and chromosomal analysis (karyotyping) is then carried out. However, the majority of babies born with congenital abnormalities have no identifiable risk markers (Nicolaides et al 1992). Mass screening of all pregnant women would be the only means of discovering an affected baby in 100% of cases, but even so there are still many conditions which cannot be detected by screening. In 1975 an Ad Hoc Committee in the United States defined genetic counselling as a 'communication process which deals with the human problem associated with the occurrence, or the risk of occurrence, of a genetic disorder in a family' (Committee of Genetic Counselling 1975). The aims of the process were

- *to help parents to understand the medical facts including the diagnosis and available management;*

- *to enable the woman and her partner to understand the relevance of inheritance in relation to the disorder and the risk of recurrence;*
- *to assess the risk to them as individuals and as a family and to choose a course of action which was suitable and which they could act upon;*
- *to make the best possible adjustment to a family member with the disorder.*

(Committee of Genetic Counselling 1975; HMSO 1993)

Ultrasound Scanning

Ultrasound scanning has increased in usefulness from a pregnancy dating tool to a diagnostic agent (Proud 1995). Forty years ago the development of the 'scan' heralded a breakthrough in information about the fetus. The technique enabled trained professionals to observe and monitor the growth of the fetus(es) without interfering with the surrounding environment. Although concern has been expressed about the lack of clear research evidence to support the safe use of ultrasound scanning during pregnancy, it remains relatively unchallenged by pregnant women (Breart and Ringa 1990; Beech and Robinson 1993).

An ultrasound scan can provide a vast amount of information in addition to fetal growth and size. Abnormalities which can be determined from an ultrasound scan include neural tube defects (e.g. spina bifida, anencephaly, hydrocephalus), skeletal abnormalities (e.g. achondroplasia, osteogenesis imperfecta), cardiac defects (e.g. hypoplastic left heart, ventricular septal defect), gastrointestinal anomalies (diaphragmatic hernia, exomphalus), and the possible identification of brain cysts. In many cases of fetal abnormality the first hint of a problem is determined during the ultrasound scan.

Timing of the ultrasound scan is variable and may depend on other screening tests available within the unit. Limitations on its effectiveness depend on the skill and expertise of the operator and the quality of the equipment used. A basic ultrasound scan will offer the opportunity to confirm the gestational age and the number and viability of babies present. All women will have access to this level of scan either at their GP surgery or in the local hospital. In order to observe the baby in more detail, an anomaly scan may be performed. The anomaly scan will allow the spine and head to be observed for any obvious lesions. The level of scan required may necessitate the woman being referred to a larger hospital. In some hospitals an anomaly scan is being routinely offered to all women at 20 weeks instead of the α-fetoprotein (αFP).

By the 20-week mark, fetal growth should enable a clear view of the spinal column and major organs.

The most advanced level of ultrasound scan is currently only available in the prenatal diagnosis department of larger hospitals. In this setting the operator can detect a wide range of suspected abnormalities such as cystic hygroma. Referrals are often sent from the smaller, less well-equipped local hospitals. Experience and use of advanced equipment enables the obstetrician or ultrasonographer to accurately diagnose or confirm many of the less commonly found congenital defects (Royal College of Physicians 1989; Parry 1993b).

Nuchal Skin Thickness

Nuchal skin thickness can be observed by ultrasound scan. The purpose of measuring the nuchal fold is to determine the presence of Down's syndrome. The procedure is non-invasive and allows immediate results, but the screening process has not yet been proved conclusive (Donnenfield et al 1994).

A study by Nicolaides et al (1994a) found that 84% of babies with Down's syndrome and 4.5% of chromosomally normal babies had a nuchal skin thickness of greater than or equal to 3 mm. The study recommended that between 10 and 13 weeks a skin thickness of 3 mm in association with raised maternal age should indicate that fetal karyotyping be performed. The recommendation was made on the basis that the link could potentially identify 85% of babies affected by Down's syndrome. A false positive rate of 5% would mean that some karyotyping is performed unnecessarily.

Method

The procedure involves an ultrasound scan at 10 to 13 weeks by an experienced ultrasonographer. As discussed, the routine availability of ultrasound scanning is dependent on different levels of expertise and client choice. The medical and midwifery staff need to be aware that this type of scan is available and how to access it, particularly if referral to a larger centre is required.

Risk of procedure

The procedure does not in itself offer risks to the pregnancy. None the less, the woman and her partner should be counselled prior to the ultrasound scan in order to appreciate the wider involvement of prenatal diagnosis and the implications if there is a thickened skinfold. They should also be aware of the false positive ratios and that this is not a conclusive screening test.

Amniocentesis

Amniocentesis is performed to facilitate chromosomal studies on the fetus. A sample of amniotic fluid is withdrawn from the intrauterine environment as described below. The sample must be cultured and examined before results can be provided. This process takes between one and three weeks. Occasionally (in about 1% of cases) the cells do not grow and a repeat procedure is requested (Parry 1993b; Kohn and Moffitt 1994a). In general the procedure is undertaken between 16 and 18 weeks, but work is currently being performed as early as 10 weeks in some specialist centres (Penso et al 1990; Parry 1993b; Nicolaides et al 1994b; Shulman et al 1994).

Method

Ultrasound guidance is required to reduce the risk of damaging the baby (Royal College of Physicians 1989; Kohn and Moffitt 1994b). Having emptied her bladder, the woman is asked to lie on a couch and an abdominal palpation is performed to determine the lie and presentation of the baby. An ultrasound scan is employed to confirm the abdominal palpation, locate the placenta and to identify a pool of amniotic fluid from which the sample may be obtained. The abdomen is cleansed and, under aseptic conditions, a needle is inserted into the uterus. A local anaesthetic may be used if the woman chooses. Approximately 10–20 ml of amniotic fluid is aspirated without touching the baby. The woman and her partner can watch the procedure on the video screen of the ultrasound machine. When the needle has been withdrawn, a small dressing such as a sticking plaster is applied over the insertion site. If the woman is Rhesus negative she will require an intramuscular injection of anti-D immunoglobulin to prevent sensitisation. This can occur in women who are Rhesus negative if fetal blood cells are transferred into maternal circulation (Sweet 1991; Parry 1993b). Following the procedure the woman may be advised to rest for a short period and she should be instructed to look for vaginal bleeding or pyrexia. Abdominal cramps may predispose the bleeding. If any of these symptoms occur she should be advised to consult her doctor or midwife as soon as possible.

Risk of procedure

There is controversy in the medical world over the incidence of pregnancy loss as a result of amniocentesis. The general acceptance of a 1% risk acknowledges that an element of uncertainty does exist, but this is difficult to measure accurately (Ager and Oliver 1986; Royal College of Physicians 1989; Parry 1993b; Kohn and Moffitt 1994a). The risks include infection,

THERAPEUTIC
TERMINATION
– Antenatal Screening

abortion, fetal death, haematoma, spontaneous rupture of membranes, haemorrhage, preterm labour and rhesus iso-immunisation (Sweet 1991).

Chorionic Villus Sampling

Chorionic villus sampling (CVS) is a procedure in which a small amount of placental tissue is withdrawn for genetic analysis. CVS was introduced for the first-trimester prenatal diagnosis of genetic disease over 20 years ago. As the placenta develops from the blastocyst, the genetic makeup of the baby is revealed in the cells. In contrast to the need to wait until the second trimester before performing an amniocentesis, CVS may be undertaken after just nine completed weeks of pregnancy (Editorial 1991). For most couples an early diagnosis is important, particularly if the pregnancy is not showing (Ward 1987; Sweet 1991; Kohn and Moffitt 1994b; MRC Working Party, 1991).

Method

The cells may be obtained transabdominally or transcervically, the latter being more commonly performed in European countries outside the United Kingdom (Parry 1993b; Kohn and Moffitt 1994b). The decision on which method to use may depend on the unit policy, the position of the placenta or the preference of the doctor.

During the procedure ultrasound guidance is used to ensure that the placenta is visualised and the sample is aspirated safely. The cannula is inserted and a syringe is used to withdraw tissue. The amount of tissue aspirated depends on the test being performed; approximately 10–20 mg is required for direct chromosomal analysis, but it is necessary to obtain more (approximately 30–60 mg) for the diagnosis of beta-thalassaemia (Royal College of Physicians 1989; Sweet 1991). Post CVS the woman may be advised to rest for the remainder of the day and to avoid sexual intercourse for a week. Anti-D prophylaxis is recommended in women who are Rhesus negative and may be repeated at intervals during the remaining pregnancy (Ward 1987). Vaginal spotting is not uncommon following CVS and is not a cause for alarm but, if worried, the woman should be encouraged to contact the hospital.

Risk of procedure

Risks to the pregnancy are considered to be higher than those associated with amniocentesis. According to Ward the relative risks are threatened abortion, cervicitis or vaginitis, fibroids, rhesus sensitisation and obesity (Ward 1987). The results of two controlled trials provide information on the comparative risks of CVS versus second-trimester amniocentesis (Editorial 1991). In 1989 results from a large Canadian trial were published (Canadian Collaborative CVS-amniocentesis Clinical Trial Group 1989), followed by the European trial in 1991 (MRC Working Party 1991). The results of both trials proved to be similar in many respects. The European results indicated that women who underwent second-trimester amniocentesis had a 4.6% greater chance of achieving a successful outcome to the pregnancy. In Canada there was a difference of 1.7% in total loss rates between the two groups when all randomised women were considered (Editorial 1991).

CVS has been associated with limb defects in the newborn. Of 30,000 women tested in a twelve-month period, it was estimated that approximately 40 babies had damaged limbs (Ryan 1995). The pregnancy loss rate following CVS can be difficult to assess accurately because the rate of spontaneous miscarriage is higher in the first trimester. By the second trimester, when amniocentesis would be the preferred option, natural loss is unlikely to occur at the same rate.

Cordocentesis

Cordocentesis is a means of obtaining fetal blood cells. Initially this was performed by a method known as fetoscopy, a specialised procedure with a fetal loss rate of 3–7% (Special Report 1984). Cordocentesis is used to identify haemoglobin disorders and haemophilia. Rapid karyotyping of fetal lymphocytes is possible following detection of a malformation by ultrasound. Biopsies of the baby's liver and skin can also be obtained (Royal College of Physicians 1989; Parry 1993b). Although it is considered to be a safer technique, cordocentesis requires an experienced operator to perform the procedure. For this reason, it is not available in all hospitals (Royal College of Physicians 1989).

The procedure is carried out at 18 weeks to ensure that the baby's blood vessels are large enough for a sample to be taken. In addition to the detection of chromosome abnormalities, cordocentesis can screen for haemoglobin disorders and intrauterine infections and allows for rapid karyotyping of an ultrasound-detected malformation (Royal College of Physicians 1989; Sweet 1991; Parry 1993b). Another advantage of this method is that the blood cells do not require culture and results are available within 48 hours.

Method

The procedure is similar to that used for amniocentesis. The woman is asked to lie on a couch and ultrasound guidance is used to observe the baby during the procedure. A cannula is inserted into the uterus, avoiding the fetus and the umbilical vein is targeted close to the insertion into the placenta. Normal saline is injected to ensure that the needle has entered the vein rather than an artery. A small amount of fetal blood (less than 4 ml) is withdrawn. Following the procedure the woman is asked to rest and the baby is observed by ultrasound for a short time.

Risk of procedure

The risks following a cordocentesis are similar to those of amniocentesis and the woman should be advised to observe for signs of infection – vaginal bleeding or leakage of liquor (Parry 1993b).

Alphafetoprotein levels

Alphafetoprotein (αFP) is a fetal plasma protein produced first by the yolk sac and then by the baby's liver. αFP is present in the amniotic fluid and also in maternal serum. Although the feto-maternal circulations do not mix, it is possible for a small number of the baby's blood cells to escape into the maternal system. Unfortunately, full serum screening which avoids the need for amniocentesis or CVS is not yet available. For the moment this method of screening can only detect neural tube defects (Royal College of Physicians 1989; Sweet 1991; Parry 1993b).

In many hospitals it is now routine to offer αFP screening between 16 and 18 weeks. Where there is an open neural tube defect such as anencephaly or spina bifida (as opposed to spina bifida occult, where the lesion is closed thereby preventing escape of the protein), the level of maternal αFP will be higher because more plasma protein will have leaked into the mother's circulation.

Method

The test is a simple blood sample obtained from the mother at the appropriate gestation. It is important to have accurate knowledge of the gestation and to know how many babies are *in utero*. This is necessary because the level of αFP increases significantly after 19 weeks or if there is more than one baby. An ultrasound scan is thus regularly performed prior to the test. It is important that the parents have a clear understanding of the purpose of the blood test. At the beginning of the pregnancy blood is obtained for a variety of routine tests and the mother may not realise that this is different or has wider implications than, for example, checking her haemoglobin level. The midwife or doctor must explain the nature of the test and what the results may mean. It must be clear that a result outside the normal range does not automatically indicate an abnormal baby. False positive results are not uncommon and may depend on a number of factors.

The woman should be told when to expect the results, which is usually after a week, and the hospital should know how to contact her if a problem occurs. If the level is raised, then a repeat sample may be requested; alternatively, she may be advised to attend for an anomaly ultrasound scan. A low reading of αFP could be an indication of Down's syndrome. Following discussion with the couple an appointment may be made for genetic counselling, resulting in an amniocentesis test (Royal College of Physicians 1989; Sweet 1991; Parry 1993b; Kohn and Moffitt 1994b). Testing for increased αFP levels is still appropriate following CVS and can be timed by ultrasound scan.

Risk of procedure

The main risk of αFP testing is an inaccurate gestational age, leading to a false positive or negative result.

Biochemical Screening

Screening of maternal serum for particular biochemical markers can given an indication of the risk of Down's syndrome. Known under a variety of names (Triple Test, Bart's Test, Leeds Test or biochemical screening), the test is a safer procedure for assessing risk than an invasive test such as amniocentesis or CVS. Therefore, women who may have experienced difficulty becoming pregnant or who have a history of recurrent miscarriages can obtain some reassurance without having to undergo a more hazardous test. Prenatal screening is usually performed on the basis of raised maternal age, yet, despite the increase in risk with advancing age, most pregnancies affected with Down's syndrome are in young women (University of Leeds 1993). An increasing number of centres are offering the facility to all women in their clinics.

Basing the need to perform additional screening tests on a history of raised maternal age or a previously affected pregnancy means that younger women are going to be missed. However, women need to appreciate that the biochemical serum test is not a

replacement for amniocentesis or CVS, which may still be
recommended if there is a screen-positive result.

Method

A blood sample is obtained between 10 and 13 weeks, although this
can vary from unit to unit and some are done later. The blood is
screened for human chorionic gonadotrophin (HCG), αFP and
unconjugated oestriol. HCG is produced and secreted by the
placenta and is raised when Down's syndrome is present.
Unconjugated oestriol and αFP are reduced in affected
pregnancies. In the event of a twin pregnancy the serum marker
levels are double those of a singleton. The marker levels are
reduced in pregnancies of women with insulin-dependent diabetes
mellitus; however, by adjusting the expected levels a risk
assessment can still be made.

Interpretation of the levels is achieved by estimating the
risk of Down's syndrome from the maternal age and the marker
levels and comparing it with a fixed cut-off risk. Adjustments must
be made for maternal weight and for ethnic origin (black women
have higher αFP and HCG levels than caucasian). If the risk is
greater than the cut-off, the result is regarded as 'screen-positive'
(University of Leeds 1993).

Screening for conditions other than Down's syndrome can
be performed on the same sample. Edward's syndrome (trisomy 18)
is the second most common chromosomal anomaly after Down's
syndrome. It is associated with advanced maternal age and low
marker levels. A raised αFP can indicate neural tube defects such
as spina bifida or anencephaly, or gastro-intestinal conditions such
as exomphalus or gastroschisis.

The results can be reported within ten working days.
Screen-positive results may be telephoned or sent by facsimile to
allow adequate time for follow up arrangements to be made.
Guidance notes on interpretation of the results are sent to the
receiving doctor. These include all relevant details used to
calculate the risk. Copies may be sent to the woman on request.
For women receiving a screen-negative result there is no need for
further counselling (University of Leeds 1993).

Biochemical screening is not currently available in all
hospitals. In some units the test will be offered routinely and sent
to a separate laboratory for analysis. In other units the woman
may have no choice but to make private arrangements to have the
blood taken and sent by her GP or midwife. The cost of the test
will then be incurred by the woman.

Triple Test Plus

In addition to biochemical screening, it is now possible to assess the level of the enzyme alkaline phosphatase in maternal neutrophils (the test is also known as NAP). Women carrying a baby with Down's syndrome have more alkaline phosphatase present in their neutrophils. Unlike the other markers used in the biochemical test, NAP is not measured in serum but is detected by microscopy on a slide prepared from whole blood (University of Leeds 1993). Women who have had a previous Down's syndrome pregnancy carry an additional risk.

Infection Screening

Maternal infections such as toxoplasmosis or cytomegalovirus can present a risk to the developing fetus. The outcome may be lethal or result in severe brain damage. Unfortunately, it is not easy to determine which babies are going to suffer long-term effects from the congenital infection (Parry 1993c). Diagnosis of the affected baby can be made by cordocentesis. Since this procedure carries an element of risk to the pregnancy in itself, the possibility of increasing the risk of losing the pregnancy by undergoing cordocentesis may be considered too great by the parents.

In the case of toxoplasmosis the woman can undergo preconceptual screening to determine her immunity to the infection. If infection occurs, treatment with antibiotics will usually overcome the problem in the woman but may not be in time to protect the baby *in utero*. The infection is diagnosed from a simple blood test.

Cytomegalovirus (CMV) is an infection which particularly affects women in the childbearing years. Transmission rates during the pregnancy do not vary so damage to the fetus may occur at any time; often the maternal infection is symptomless.

ISSUES SURROUNDING THERAPEUTIC TERMINATION OF PREGNANCY

The aim of prenatal screening is to identify those women who are carrying a baby with a handicapping condition. To many prospective parents, however, prenatal tests are interpreted as a means of confirming the health of the baby. Very few undergo the screening expecting to be told that their baby has a severe abnormality (Farrant 1985; Daker and Bobrow 1993; Stewart and Dent 1994). Ultrasound scanning expecting is seen as a screening test which confirms the perfect baby to the willing parents (Proud 1995).

The appreciation of the tests available and the implications of those tests may be related to attitude. The age of the pregnant woman may influence her understanding of the potential problems which screening can reveal. Alternatively her view of termination of pregnancy may affect how willing she is to accept screening (Green 1995). Younger women, particularly teenagers, may fall into the category of women who never expect to hear 'bad' news. Indeed, their knowledge of reproductive life may be very limited.

Further to a diagnosis of an abnormality for which there is no treatment, the woman and her partner have two options: they can either use the information to prepare for the birth of a handicapped child or they can have the pregnancy terminated (Green 1995). It is essential that the couple have the opportunity to discuss every aspect of the problem with the appropriate experts, are enabled to express their wishes and are given every opportunity to make an informed choice (Joint Study Group on Fetal Abnormalities 1989). In the case of a multiple pregnancy the discovery of a fetal abnormality in one of the babies will present the woman with a very difficult situation. In this instance, as with all women undergoing investigative tests it is vital that she understands the implications of each test and what it may reveal. There are ethical issues involved with terminating a pregnancy with a known healthy fetus (Lewis and Bryson 1988).

Choosing to terminate a pregnancy is never easy even when the reason is not termed 'therapeutic'. Undergoing the stress of attending a hospital or clinic, making arrangements, dealing with the routine aspects of normal life, trying to ensure privacy, and talking over and over about the options all add to the difficulty of the decision. For many women who undergo a termination on the grounds of impaired mental health, the strongest emotion is likely to be one of relief (Broome 1984). Green and colleagues studied the reaction of 1824 pregnant women's reactions to termination. They discovered that the most sympathetic response to termination occurred when the mother's health was in serious danger (97%). Eighty-four per cent of women felt that termination should be legally available where there was a *strong* chance that the baby would be abnormal. The inclination dropped to 50% where the likelihood of a handicap being present was less certain. The least sympathy was for those women who were married and did not want the pregnancy (37%) (Green et al 1993).

For these reasons the woman needs help to talk about how she would cope with an 'affected' child, the implications of the condition and the long-term prognosis. Religion may play an important role in the decision-making process and she should be encouraged to talk as widely as she feels necessary. The conflict of choice is not easy. In the majority of cases (although by no means all) the woman will have a partner who must also be considered. Coming to terms with being in control of destiny is a heavy responsibility for couples to deal with. The sensitive nature of the abortion issue is exacerbated by the debate over the definition of a fetal abnormality. The clause in the Abortion Act states that it is necessary that

> *there is a substantial risk that if the child were born it would suffer from such physical or mental abnormalities as to be seriously handicapped.*
>
> (Department of Health 1967)

But what does seriously handicapped mean? Christian Action Research and Education are a group concerned that if a minor abnormality such as cleft palate is diagnosed on ultrasound the pregnancy is being terminated. This minor physical defect, which is correctable after birth, is certainly not life-threatening (Field 1992). Identification of a minor problem should be an indicator only and should encourage the medical staff to observe the baby closely for a major defect. It should not be a reason to terminate the pregnancy.

Meanwhile, the pregnancy will have continued in the period of waiting for results. It may still be possible for the prospective mother to conceal her pregnancy if she chooses, but she cannot hide it from herself. Fetal movements are felt between 16 and 18 weeks. Many women undergoing prenatal testing will already have felt their baby move:

> *Once the woman declares, even to herself, that she has felt the baby move, that is that ... once felt it cannot be unfelt.*
>
> (Katz Rothman 1988)

In addition, the ultrasound scan will have provided real-time pictures of a living, moving baby. This image is likely to have been shared with her partner, and possibly with some members of the extended family. With a healthy baby the routine ultrasound scan provides early evidence that the pregnancy is more than morning sickness and tiredness; it also makes the whole event a reality for the partner who is not experiencing the altering body image or symptoms of pregnancy. The journey home may be spent discussing the physical characteristics and the behaviour of the baby on screen or looking again at the photograph from the machine. For the couple who receive bad news at the scan appointment or who have the scan specifically for a potential problem, the period

THERAPEUTIC
TERMINATION
– Other Issues

afterwards will be very different. Their conversation will focus on the implications of the diagnosis and the scheduling of further tests, if required. Evidence of the baby does not help the decision-making process at this stage, particularly if the pregnancy has been difficult to achieve, possibly following a prolonged period of infertility or recurrent miscarriages.

The decision regarding a termination of pregnancy for fetal abnormality is made following a series of prenatal tests. Referral for these tests may come from the woman herself, her GP or the obstetrician. Consideration has been given to the particular tests currently available in the United Kingdom, but referral is not always acceptable to women and it is imperative that staff understand the implications involved in the referral.

Undergoing Prenatal Screening Tests

The prime objective of genetic screening is to reduce the overall burden of a disorder within a population (Daker and Bobrow 1993); the same could be said of all prenatal screening tests. The discovery of a disorder or potential handicap at an early gestation means either treatment may be given as soon after birth as possible or, if appropriate and acceptable, the pregnancy may be terminated. The decision about which tests should be performed, and when, is a medical one. The decision about whether to have these tests rests with the woman. If she decides against prenatal screening, the staff providing maternity care have a duty to respect her wishes and support that decision. It is essential that she is able to make a fully informed choice and the midwife, GP, obstetrician and associated specialists must play their role in ensuring this is the case (HMSO 1993). Where there are cultural, religious or ethical reasons, both the woman and her partner must be supported in reaching the correct decision for them. Fear exists that focusing on genetic problems associated with particular ethnic groups will be considered racist, but the real discrimination occurs in failing to provide the necessary medical service with access to information and interpreters (Royal College of Physicians 1989).

Certain tests provide immediate results and lead to certain practical issues. Breaking bad news to someone is difficult enough in a consulting room or in the ward area. An ultrasound room is not usually designed to allocate space for sitting and talking about the findings in great detail. But the alternative may be the waiting room or the corridor outside. Consideration has to be given to the best place to talk after the scan and how to inform medical staff of the results. With investigations which are processed through a laboratory the situation is more controlled. The doctor has a clear idea of the length of time involved in receiving a result and can make arrangements accordingly. There may be a policy of informing clients by telephone or via the GP, neither of which offers the same continuity as a personal appointment. The couple may be instructed to interpret 'no news' as 'good news', but a timescale for expected results needs to be given. If there is a possibility of a false positive result the woman ought to be informed rather than assuming her baby is in trouble.

Ultrasound scanning gives immediate results. If the operator is not a doctor, a local agreement should be in place that describes how the results will be given to the woman. It would be naive to imagine that the woman and her partner would miss unspoken signals of bad news – a sudden silence in the room, a shift in body language and so forth can all indicate a problem. The need for a doctor to break the news may be dictated by hospital policy, but the scan operator needs guidelines as well. At a minimum these guidelines must explain how far to go in describing a potential problem. If the scan is being performed for a known risk such as raised αFP, then the doctor should be present. Kenyon's retrospective study of women following therapeutic termination found that some objected to being told the diagnosis in front of everyone in the ultrasound room (Kenyon 1988).

A poor outcome from prenatal screening indicates to the parents that a discussion on the future of their baby is inevitable. The solution to most abnormalities found on ultrasound screening is termination of the pregnancy. Understanding the various tests is important for the woman and her partner. They need to know what the test will and will not tell them and the inherent risks. Couples need information, not only on the nature of the test, but on the range of ability or disability and prognosis which may attach to specific conditions and about the way they may feel having undergone a termination of pregnancy (Downe 1994).

They also need reassurance that a termination is not necessary even if an abnormality is identified. Finally, they need to appreciate that the test can also provide positive news in respect of confirming a normal baby (Katz Rothman 1988; Parry 1993a). The diagnosis must be clearly explained to them as frequently as required. Physical and mental space to accept the news must be given and the woman should never be expected to return to a crowded waiting room (Mander 1994). If the woman is alone and wishes her partner to be contacted, the staff should attend to this immediately. Further to the ultrasound scan it may be necessary to recommend other investigations and counselling.

Repetition may be necessary in order for the news to sink in. Other family members may also be involved. It may not be possible for the couple to reach a consensus decision, or they may change their mind over a matter of days or hours (Stewart and Dent 1994). The opportunity to return to the hospital and talk further with the counsellor, doctor or midwife should always be available and knowledge of how to access this service should be given to all women who attend.

The development of screening tests for fetal abnormality seems to point the way towards a world without handicap. The belief that the pursuit of perfection is somehow attainable and that the identification of abnormalities means that they can somehow be eliminated is not justified. Proud suggests that

> *The idea that a perfect baby is somehow the only acceptable outcome of a pregnancy is one which parents, midwives and obstetricians have come to expect.*
>
> (Proud 1995)

Katz Rothman argues that the use of prenatal diagnosis and termination of an affected pregnancy directly affects the area of research into the diagnosed abnormality. Using Tay-Sachs disease as an example she examines how the isolation of the parents imposed by prenatal discovery rather than the birth of children afflicted with this lethal condition deters basic research. No longer faced with a ward of suffering children and with limited resources available for research, doctors do not have the same impetus to find a cure for this particular disease. Those women who slip through the net, miss the screening or elect to continue the pregnancy, quickly find themselves parents without a support network. But the answer is not to stop the development of prenatal screening. As Katz Rothman argues:

> *It certainly seems very wrong to [reject the technology] ... in order to have babies around to experiment on to find cures.*
>
> (Katz Rothman 1988)

Positive news following prenatal diagnosis is not an absolute guarantee of a perfect baby. The investigations performed will have concentrated on specific malformations or genetic disorders. Various problems can still occur, for example cleft palate and/or hare lip. If, as Downe asks, the woman then has a baby with an undetected problem, 'how do they deal with the situation, having not undergone the psychological preparation of the "what-if" scenario?' (Downe 1994). There is no easy answer: shock and bewilderment will surface as, having been lulled into a false sense of security, the woman may become angry with the nearest member of staff, or withdraw into herself and away from the baby. The staff may have warned her of the limitations of the specific test, but this may not have been appreciated. Communication is a key factor in the care of all women in childbirth; particular challenges are presented by those who experience perinatal deaths.

In 1989 a special report on recognition and management of fetal abnormalities by members of the joint study group on fetal abnormalities stated:

> *It is the duty of the team involved in antenatal diagnosis not only to work closely together so as to create a rational plan of management but to communicate sympathetically and comprehensively with the parents.*
> (Joint Study Group on Fetal Abnormalities 1989)

Methods for Late Termination of Pregnancy

The reasons for performing a termination of pregnancy after the first trimester can be varied. Ending a wanted and planned pregnancy for fetal abnormality will be a traumatic experience for the parents, a fact which staff need to remember when expecting the couple to help in the decision-making process. The complications and maternal mortality rate of induced abortions rise with increasing gestation, so it is important to minimize delay in carrying out the procedure once the decision is made (Savage 1990). In completing the abortion notification form, implemented in 1982, medical staff are not required to identify how the termination was achieved. The omission of this information means that the use of intra-amniotic or extra-amniotic methods is unknown in official statistics.

In the United Kingdom a medical method of termination is employed, commonly prostaglandin instillation into the space between the membranes and myometrium via the cervix. A Foley catheter is inserted transcervically and a solution of prostaglandin is administered. The action is prolonged (up to 14 hours) and intravenous syntocinon may be prescribed to potentiate the action of the prostaglandin. Alternatively, prostaglandin pessaries may be administered by the vaginal route.

The possibility of delivering a live baby is to be considered and the mother should be aware of this. Previously, urea was administered by intracardiac injection to the fetus under ultrasound guidance; the effect of this was to ensure that the baby was not born alive. The withdrawal from pharmacies of the 'drug' urea has meant that this method is no longer available. Signs of life in the pre-viable baby may present ethical issues for the staff involved. Sensitive handling is required when discussing the management of the baby.

Guidelines for care can assist at this time. When the decision has been made to terminate the pregnancy and the baby is born alive, the question of resuscitation may be raised. It is inappropriate to actively resuscitate a baby after the pregnancy has been deliberately terminated. Parents may have a misconception about how the baby will be treated: stories of aborted fetuses being abandoned in the sluice room or flushed away have led to concern. The parents have a right to know the condition of the baby at the time of delivery; they may wish to be involved in caring for the baby until signs of life are no longer present. Voicing their concerns may be difficult for the couple and the staff may need to be proactive over this issue. Explaining clearly what will happen to the baby post delivery is important. The baby should be handled carefully and wrapped in a cot sheet and a blanket. The delicate tissues will bruise easily and the skin may tear. As the mother will require attention it may be difficult for the midwife to devote her time to the baby. If the parents do not wish to see and hold the baby he or she can be placed in a small Moses basket or the hospital cot and kept in the room. If the parents object to the baby's presence close to them, the midwife will have to find an alternative such as an unoccupied delivery room. Other members of staff need to be aware of the baby's presence and attention should be given to visiting staff, particularly those conducting an antenatal class tour of the delivery suite for expectant mothers. Walking into a room where a baby is being given terminal care or is already deceased will cause immense distress to anyone who is ill-prepared. The parents should be informed when the baby dies.

Where signs of life are present, a legal responsibility exists for the parents to register the baby. In effect, the baby becomes a live birth and a neonatal death. To staff, registration may appear unnecessarily cruel, but it is still required. The temptation to ignore the life signs or legal requirements may be strong, particularly as the parents are unlikely to think of it. However, by choosing not to recognise the baby as a live birth, staff may be denying the parents the opportunity to acknowledge their son or daughter as a legally recorded person. In the future it may become very important to them to remember their child by looking at the birth certificate. In addition, the process of grieving may be enhanced by the necessity of registering the details. The purpose of providing photographs of the baby is to give the parents a positive memory of the baby; a certificate from the Registrar's Office may have the same effect.

The Health Professional's Attitude to Termination

Gynaecology nurses

Ongoing support and guidance following the decision to terminate the pregnancy are critical to the care of the woman. Actually providing that care may present moral dilemmas for the doctor, nurse or midwife involved. Depending on the gestation and local policy, the woman may be cared for in the gynaecology ward, the antenatal ward or the delivery suite. Therefore, the issues surrounding conscientious objections on the grounds of moral, ethical or religious beliefs can arise in any of these locations. Webb studied the attitudes of gynaecology nurses towards termination of pregnancy in social circumstances (i.e. for reasons other than fetal abnormality). She discovered that the nurses had negative attitudes towards women undergoing termination of pregnancy and were quite condemnatory of them (Webb 1985). This negativity was more significant the longer the nurses had been in the post and the closer they were to the practical side of the job. Nurses stressed the discomfort they felt in dealing with the physical care of the baby when he or she was delivered. The study was published in 1985 in a climate of economic depression and the nurses involved had not elected to work in gynaecology as their first career choice — a fact which highlights the importance of ensuring that the nurses are comfortable in their knowledge and ability to deal with these situations (Webb 1985).

Historically, gynaecology nurses have provided excellent care to women undergoing medical or surgical procedures, while midwives on a delivery suite have looked after women in childbirth. The expansion of day surgeries to include surgical termination of pregnancy, however, has meant that a woman undergoing this procedure may never enter a gynaecology ward. In addition, the hospital may not perform medical terminations, that is those later than 12 weeks, which are fewer in number and may be referred to another hospital contracted to provide this service. If this situation exists in a hospital, the nurses on the gynaecology ward may have no experience of caring for women having a termination.

Privacy is also important. There is an argument against shutting women into side-rooms as this may enhance their impression of being different and create more isolation. It is less easy to communicate with staff when one is closed off from them. Delivery suites are designed with the purpose of allowing labouring women the privacy of their own room, and staff are accustomed to working in this environment and behave differently from general ward management. As Stewart points out, there is a

THERAPEUTIC TERMINATION - Other Issues

need to be sensitive to issues of privacy and dignity (Stewart and Dent 1994).

Obstetricians

The views of obstetricians regarding therapeutic termination were surveyed in 1980 when amniocentesis and maternal serum alphafetoprotein screening were relatively new techniques. The survey was repeated in 1993 and revealed some changes in the attitudes of obstetricians towards prenatal diagnosis. The original study was only partially reported in 1985 but it gave an indication of the different agendas of the professional and the client. In the main the professionals saw the aim of prenatal diagnosis as the detection of fetal abnormalities, while women wanted the reassurance that the baby was perfect.

A major change in the two surveys was the proportion of obstetricians who required the client to agree to termination if an abnormality was found on the amniocentesis. Seventy-five per cent of doctors in 1980 refused to proceed with the investigation without this undertaking; in 1993 34% were still insisting on the woman making the decision in advance of the test.

Late termination was considered by more obstetricians in the later study, although few were prepared to go as far as the law now permitted. Only 13% would recommend termination for Down's syndrome after 24 weeks (Green 1995). The diagnosis is sufficient for doctors to consider that the abnormality merits termination earlier in the pregnancy, and a lot of resources are being spent on diagnosing the condition. Yet obstetricians expressed concern that it does not fulfil the criteria for late termination. The conflict lies in the interpretation of the words 'serious' and 'substantive' in the Abortion Act, which are not clearly defined. Green suggests that clarification is required with some urgency (Green 1995).

Midwives

The midwife's relationship with a pregnant woman extends to the unborn baby as well. Concern for the safety and well-being of the baby must be maintained throughout the pregnancy. Close monitoring of the fetal condition is a critical element of the midwife's responsibility and must be carried out in accordance with the Midwives Rules (UKCC 1993). Sometimes, following a diagnosis of fetal abnormality, the midwife may feel compelled to create a distinction of care. As Opoku suggests, this distinction occurs because midwives believe that they have a duty beyond the care of the pregnant mother (Opoku 1993).

Is the answer, then, to divorce the midwife from women undergoing second-trimester termination of pregnancy? The woman undergoing a therapeutic termination of pregnancy may have a limited choice in where she is cared for, owing to the fact that 'social' terminations are carried out on the gynaecology ward. This, as Jowett observed, may be the

> *final insult and condemnation from the profession that, after all the interest and support antenatally, at the time of termination the midwives are absent?*

(Jowett 1989)

Kenyon agrees with this view. In her study of the needs of women undergoing therapeutic termination, she discovered that women appreciated the presence of a midwife, arguing that the midwife is more accustomed to coping with the stresses involved in this type of labour (Kenyon 1988).

Thus the midwife may appear to be the most appropriate person to provide care, but what if she or he has a conscientious objection to termination of pregnancy? The Abortion Act of 1967 addressed the issue of conscientious objections in Section 4:

> *Subject to subsection (2) of this section no person shall be under any duty, whether by contract or any statutory or other legal requirements to participate in any treatment authorised in this Act to which he (or she) has a conscientious objection: provided that in legal proceedings the burden of proof of conscientious objection shall rest on the person claiming to rely on it.*

(Department of Health 1967)

But the wording of the Act gives no rights to the nurse or midwife to withdraw based on the individual circumstances of the case (Field 1992). The expectation is that the nurse or midwife will have decided upon their attitude towards termination at the beginning of their career. In some situations this may be so, but for many others their attitudes will be formed over a period of time and their response may vary according to the circumstances. Just as Green discovered that pregnant women's attitudes towards termination changed depending on the reason for the request, so it can be with nurses and midwives; the fact that a termination is being carried out for a fetal abnormality may be more acceptable than a contraception failure (Blain 1993). With the increase in direct-entry courses for student midwives without a previous nursing qualification, the experience may be given little advance thought. As a result, the attitudinal issues surrounding pregnancy loss must be considered within the midwifery curriculum. Gynaecology nurses and midwives should be available to provide

THERAPEUTIC TERMINATION – Other Issues

advice and appropriate counselling and to help the students and new midwives deal with these issues up front. By law, all nurses, midwives and health visitors are subject to the authority of the United Kingdom Central Council (UKCC). In the Code of Professional Conduct the UKCC states that the nurse or midwife must 'report to an appropriate person or authority, at the earliest possible time, any conscientious objection which may be relevant to your professional practice' (UKCC 1992).

Women do perceive staff attitudes towards them; nurses and midwives need to show sympathy and understanding, both of which may prove difficult if they are unable to justify the woman's actions (Blain 1993). Doctors who have an objection to termination of pregnancy ensure that they involve colleagues who do not share their concern in the management of the woman, and Jowett advocates that nurses and midwives follow this lead. She argues that the situation is rarely an emergency, so planning for care is feasible. The discovery of a significant abnormality where the parents make a decision to end the pregnancy may include the request to do so immediately. Usually this will be the choice of the couple rather than a medical emergency, but invariably the delivery suite will be asked to adapt to the situation at short notice.

The Supervisor of Midwives is concerned with the safety in practice and care and should support the midwife as a 'colleague, counsellor and advisor' (UKCC 1994). As prenatal diagnostic work increases, so does the number of therapeutic terminations of pregnancy. Even when the hospital does not carry out the advanced screening tests, the woman may choose to have the procedure performed locally. Therefore staff may find themselves adapting to the needs of clients not previously catered for and the issue of a conscientious objection may suddenly become a contentious one. Staff may be unsure who to approach, and the less experienced or newly qualified nurse or midwife may be particularly vulnerable in this situation.

A candidate who has applied for a post may ask whether termination of pregnancy is conducted and decide for himself or herself about taking a job there. Alternatively, the interviewer may include the information as a general view of the work of the unit. Care must be taken to ensure that the candidate is not discriminated against over a conscientious objection. The knowledge that a member of staff does not wish to be involved in this type of work should be used for planning purposes and staffing the area on particular days.

So where does the answer lie? Are women receiving substandard care because the midwife or nurse disagrees with their choice (Opoku 1993)? If so, the nursing and midwifery management need to identify and address the issues. Assessment of the particular skills of the staff to ensure that there is no requirement on those who do have a genuine objection to this type of work having to compromise their beliefs is paramount. The day-to-day management of the workload may preclude absolute guarantees, but a sensitive approach which shows understanding and appreciation may go a long way in reaching a compromise in troubled times.

REFERENCES

Ager RP & Oliver RWA (1986) The risks of midtrimester amniocentesis. In *Biological Materials Analysis Research Unit*. Salford, University of Salford.

Altman DG & Hytten FE (1993) Assessment of fetal size and fetal growth. In (I Chalmers, M Enkin & MJNC Keirse, eds) *Effective Care in Pregnancy and Childbirth*, pp 411–418. Oxford, Oxford University Press.

Beech BL & Robinson J (1993) Ultrasound??? Unsound. *AIMS Journal* 5: 3.

Blain S (1993) Abortion: No middle ground. *Nursing Standard* 7: 47.

Breart G & Ringa V (1990) Routine or selective ultrasound scanning. In (M Hall, ed.) *Baillière's Clinical Obstetrics and Gynaecology: Antenatal Care*, vol 4, no. 1, pp 45–63. London, Baillière Tindall.

Broome A (1984) Abortion counselling. *Nursing Mirror* 158. 19.

Canadian Collaborative CVS-Amniocentesis Clinical Trial Group (1989) Multicentre randomised clinical trial of chorion villus sampling and amniocentesis: First report. *Lancet* i: 1–6.

Committee of Genetic Counselling (ad hoc) (1975) Genetic counselling. *American Journal of Human Genetics* 27: 240–242.

Daker M & Bobrow M (1993) Screening for genetic disease and fetal anomaly during pregnancy. In (I Chalmers, M Enkin & MJNC Keirse, eds) *Effective Care in Pregnancy and Childbirth*, pp 366–381. Oxford, Oxford University Press.

Department of Health, *Abortion Act*. 1967. London, HMSO.

Department of Health (1993) Reviewing antenatal care. In *Changing Childbirth*, pp 19–22. London, HMSO.

Donnenfield AE, Carlson RE, Palomaki GE, Librezzi RJ, Wiener S & Platt LD (1994) Prospective multicentre study of second-trimester nuchal skinfold thickness in unaffected and Down syndrome pregnancies. *Obstetrics and Gynaecology* 84: 844–847.

Downe S (1994) Screening for genetic abnormalities: Risks and benefits. *British Journal of Midwifery* 2: 406–407.

Editorial (1991) Chorionic villus sampling: Valuable addition or dangerous alternative? *Lancet* 337: 1513–1515.

Enkin M, Keirse MJNC & Chalmers I (1990) Effective care in pregnancy and childbirth. In (I Chalmers, M Enkin & MJNC Keirse, eds) *A Guide to Effective Care in Pregnancy and Childbirth*, pp 1–3. Oxford, Oxford University Press.

Farrant W (1985) Who's for amniocentesis? The politics of prenatal screening. In (H Homans, ed.) *The Sexual Politics of Reproducing.* London, Gower Medical Publishing.

Field D (1992) The 'conscience clause' and moral dilemmas. *Senior Nurse* **12**: 18–21.

Green JM (1995) Obstetricians' views on prenatal diagnosis and termination of pregnancy: 1980 compared with 1993. *British Journal of Obstetrics and Gynaecology* **102**: 228–232.

Green JM, Snowdon C & Statham H (1993) Pregnant women's attitude to abortion and prenatal screening. *Journal of Reproductive and Infant Psychology* **11**: 31–39.

HMSO (1993) *Population Needs and Genetic Services: An Outline Guide.* London, HMSO.

Joint Study Group on Fetal Abnormalities (1989) Recognition and management of fetal abnormalities. *Archives of Disease in Childhood* **64**: 971–976.

Jowett SG (1989) Therapeutic abortion – who cares? *Midwives' Chronicle and Nursing Notes* October: 334.

Katz Rothman B (1988) Making choices. In *The Tentative Pregnancy*, pp 49–85. London, Pandora Press.

Kenyon S (1988) Support after termination for fetal abnormality. *Midwives' Chronicle and Nursing Notes* June: 190–191.

Kohn I & Moffitt PL (1994a) Appendix A: Managing problem pregnancies. In *Pregnancy Loss: A Silent Sorrow*, pp 236–250. London, Hodder Headline.

Kohn I & Moffitt PL (1994b) Stillborn and newborn death. In *Pregnancy Loss: A Silent Sorrow*, pp 90–105. London, Hodder Headline.

Lewis E & Bryson EM (1988) Management of perinatal loss of a twin. *British Medical Journal* **297**: 1321–1323.

Mander R (1994) Features of loss in childbearing. In *Loss and Bereavement in Childbearing*, pp 35–55. Oxford, Blackwell Scientific Publications.

MRC Working Party (1991) Medical Research Council European trial of chorionic villus sampling. *Lancet* **337**: 1491–1499.

Newton C & Walker G (1994) Down's syndrome: The need for audit. *British Journal of Midwifery* **2**: 409–411.

Nicolaides KH, Brizot MdeL & Snijders RJM (1994a) Fetal nuchal translucency: Ultrasound screening for fetal trisomy in the first trimester of pregnancy. *British Journal of Obstetrics and Gynaecology* **101**: 782–786.

Nicolaides K, Brizot MdeL, Patel F & Snijders R (1994b) Comparison of chorionic villus sampling and amniocentesis for fetal karyotyping at 10 to 13 weeks gestation. *Lancet* **344**: 435–439.

Nicolaides KH, Snijders RJM, Gosden CM, Berry C & Campbell S (1992) Ultrasonographically detectable markers of fetal chromosomal abnormalities. *Lancet* **340**: 704–707.

OPCS (1986) Ethnic minority populations in Great Britain. In *Population Trends*. London, HMSO.

Opoku D (1993) Midwives' attitudes to abortion. *British Journal of Midwifery* **1**: 62.

Parry V (1993a) Routine tests. In *The Antenatal Testing Handbook*, pp 22–39. London, Pan Books.

Parry V (1993b) Ultrasound. In *The Antenatal Testing Handbook*, pp 87–100. London, Pan Books.

Parry V (1993c) Testing for toxoplasmosis. In *The Antenatal Testing Handbook*, pp 147–155. London, Pan Books.

Pembrey ME (1987) The impact of DNA analysis on fetal diagnosis. *Baillière's Clinical Obstetrics and Gynaecology*, vol 1, no. 3, pp 569–589. London, Baillière Tindall.

Penso C, Sandstrom MM, Garber M-F, Ladoulis M, Stryker JM & Benacerraf BB (1990) Early amniocentesis: report of 407 cases with neonatal follow up. *Obstetrics and Gynaecology* **76**: 1032–1036.

Proud J (1995) Ethics and obstetric ultrasound. *British Journal of Midwifery* **3**: 79–82.

Royal College of Physicians (1989) *Prenatal Diagnosis and Genetic Screening*, pp 14–22. London, Royal College of Physicians.

Ryan S (1995) Test for pregnant women causes wave of birth defects. *Sunday Times*, 12 March.

Savage W (1990) Late induced abortion. *Contemporary Review of Obstetrics and Gynaecology* **2**: 163–170.

Shulman LP, Elias S, Phillips OP, Grevengood C, Dungar JS & Simpson JL (1994) Amniocentesis performed at 14 weeks gestation or earlier: Comparison with first trimester transabdominal chorionic villus sampling. *Obstetrics and Gynaecology* **83**: 543–548.

Smith DK & Marteau TM (1995) Detecting fetal abnormality: Serum screening and fetal anomaly scans. *British Journal of Midwifery* **2**: 406–407.

Special Report (1984) The status of fetoscopy and fetal tissue sampling. *Prenatal Diagnosis* **4**: 79–81.

Stewart A & Dent A (1994) Lost beginnings: When pregnancy ends before birth. In (A Stewart & A Dent, eds) *At A Loss*, pp 13–50. London, Baillière Tindall.

Sweet B (1991) Antenatal investigation of maternal and fetal wellbeing. In (B Sweet, ed.) *Maye's Midwifery*, 11th edn reprint, pp 158–169. London, Baillière Tindall.

Tew M (1995) The practices of attendants before birth. In (M Tew, ed.) *Safer Childbirth*, pp 86–194. London, Chapman and Hall.

UKCC (1992) Code of Professional Conduct, Section 8. United Kingdom Central Council for Nursing, Midwifery and Hospital Visiting.

UKCC (1993) Responsibility and sphere of practice. *Midwives' Rules* **40**: 1. United Kingdom Central Council for Nursing, Midwifery and Hospital Visiting.

UKCC (1994) Supervisors of Midwives. In *The Midwives' Code of Practice*, p 17. United Kingdom Central Council for Nursing, Midwifery and Health Visiting.

University of Leeds (1993) *Screening for Down's syndrome*. Information booklet. University of Leeds Institute of Epidemiology.

Wald N (1984) *Antenatal and Neonatal Screening*. Oxford, Oxford University Press.

Ward RHT (1987) Techniques of chorionic villus sampling. *Baillière's Clinical Obstetrics and Gynaecology*, vol 1, no. 3, pp 489–512. London, Baillière Tindall.

Webb C (1985) Nurses' attitude to therapeutic abortion. *Nursing Times* 81: 44–47.

Chapter Five

Stillbirth

'Stillborn child' means a child which has issued forth from its mother after the twenty-fourth week of pregnancy and which did not at any time after being completely expelled from its mother breathe or show any other signs of life, and the expression 'stillbirth' shall be used accordingly (section 41).
(Stillbirth (Definition) Act 1992)

The definition of stillbirth in the Births and Deaths Registration Act 1953 was altered by the Stillbirth Act 1992. Previously defined as a pregnancy which had lasted 28 weeks or more, the change reduced the age of viability to 24 weeks.

The registration of stillbirths was introduced in England and Wales in 1928. At that time the stillbirth rate was 41 per 1000 births. This remained constant until 1935 when a gradual decrease occurred until 1939 followed by a rapid fall until it reached an impressive 22.6 per 1000 births in 1950. Scotland has recorded stillbirths since 1939 and the rate started to fall after 1940 (Tew 1995). In England and Wales between 1989 and 1990 the stillbirth rate (stillbirths per 1000 total births) fell from 4.7 to 4.6, again the lowest rate ever recorded (Stillbirth (Definitions) Act 1992).

The terminology surrounding stillbirths can be confusing. A differentiation is made between those babies who died before labour had commenced and those whose demise occurred during the intrapartum period. When a stillbirth occurs during the pregnancy, it is referred to as an intrauterine death; diagnosis of the death may follow a routine antenatal visit or because the mother presented with a particular complaint, for example vaginal bleeding or lack of fetal movements. Suspicions of complications are confirmed, usually by ultrasound scan technique, and the labour is induced at a time agreed with the couple. At birth the baby may have a macerated appearance which the parents should be prepared for. In the case of an intrapartum death the baby dies during the labour and is also known as a "fresh" stillbirth; the event will inevitably be shocking for everybody involved and staff will have to deal with their own emotions at the same time as the parents are in the acute phase of the loss.

The causes of death can be maternal or fetal problems, but in many cases no cause of death is determined. In 1990 there were 3256 stillbirths; of these 31% had neither a main fetal or main maternal condition recorded.

CAUSES OF STILLBIRTH: MATERNAL FACTORS

Despite the decrease in perinatal mortality figures since 1976, women with a previous stillbirth or a fetal abnormality or who are over 35 years of age are at an increased risk of suffering a stillbirth (Table 5.1) (Beischer and Mackay 1988). Maternal age is becoming more significant as more women are waiting later to have babies (Parry 1993).

Existing medical conditions in the mother such as renal disease or hypertensive disorders contribute significantly to perinatal mortality. Although the prevalence of heart disease in the Western world is no greater than 1%, it continues to have an impact on the rate of maternal mortality. If the mother suffers from a particular medical disorder, there may be placental insufficiency and the baby's growth can then be affected, resulting in severe problems and occasionally stillbirth (Alberman 1989).

Diabetes Mellitus

Diabetes mellitus is a medical condition in which the pancreas fails to produce sufficient insulin for the body. Insulin is required for the storage and the consumption of glucose, enabling the liver and muscles to store glucose and the tissues to burn it. The latter fails to occur when there is insufficient insulin and this leads to an accumulation of glucose in the bloodstream (Sweet 1991a). Gestational diabetes mellitus is defined as glucose intolerance during pregnancy and the diagnosis is based on an abnormal oral glucose tolerance test (Hunter 1994a).

Table 5.1 Stillbirths in the UK: numbers and rates per 1000 total births, by maternal age (Stillbirth (Definition) Act 1992)

All ages (no.)	<20 years (no.)	20–24 years (no.)	25–29 years (no.)	30–34 years (no.)	35 and over (no.)
2,762 (4.4%)	317 (6.0%)	706 (4.3%)	903 (4.0%)	523 (3.9%)	313 (6.3%)

Thirty years ago the risk of diabetes mellitus in the pregnant woman carried a high perinatal mortality rate. In the 1990s tighter control of this condition has reduced the risk considerably. What is unclear is whether this is a direct result of better control of diabetes mellitus or due to the total programme of care involved (Hunter 1994b). The incidence of insulin-dependent diabetes mellitus is in the order of 1 in 500 pregnancies; non-insulin-dependent diabetes mellitus is less frequent (Maresh 1990).

In 1980 the World Health Organisation defined diabetes mellitus as a random blood sugar level greater than 11 mmol/l (200 mg/dl) or a fasting value of greater than 8 mmol/l (140 mg/dl), in the presence of symptoms of diabetes (polyuria, polydipsia, ketoacidosis) (Hunter 1994b). The procedure for an abnormal oral glucose tolerance test varies. The World Health Organisation recommends the use of 75 mg of glucose rather than 50 mg. Abnormal findings following the ingestion of the glucose would show a fasting blood sugar greater than 7.0 mmol/l (129 mg/dl) and a two-hour blood sugar greater than 10.0 mmol/l (190 mg/dl) (Sweet 1991a; Hunter 1994b).

Women with pre-existing diabetes mellitus should be encouraged to consult their physician to plan the pregnancy and to try to ensure optimal health immediately before conception. The decision about when to become pregnant may be difficult and expert advice would be required to enable a couple to determine the risks involved and the likelihood of those risks increasing if the pregnancy is delayed (Hunter 1994a).

The risks to the fetus depend on the maternal condition. The woman whose diabetes is kept under control and who attends for antenatal care has a better chance of progressing to the third trimester and a delivery at term. Antenatal care is aimed at detecting a deterioration in the maternal condition which may present as hypertension, polyhydramnios, vascular complications (retinopathy), renal complications or macrosomia in the baby. An appropriate medical response is required immediately (Sweet 1991a; Maresh 1990; Hunter 1994a).

An alternative view of diabetes mellitus in pregnancy is offered by Hunter and Keirse, who argue that the treatment of gestational diabetes mellitus with insulin has not led to a decrease in the incidence of perinatal loss and that it has created a potential to do more harm than good. An abnormal glucose tolerance test is associated with an increased incidence of macrosomic infants, but the majority of such babies will be delivered to mothers with a normal glucose tolerance test. They recommend that glucose tolerance testing should cease to be used for other than research purposes and that obstetric research be concentrated into the 'true risk, if any, associated with sub-diabetic degrees of hyperglycaemia during pregnancy' (Hunter 1994a).

Rhesus Incompatibility

Haemolytic disease of the newborn (HDN) as a result of Rhesus (Rh) incompatibility is virtually unheard of today. In the same way as tuberculosis was once regarded as a common and often lethal disease, the incidence of HDN has reduced in incidence and importance as a cause of mortality (Fairweather 1989). In the decades leading up to the mid-1960s, Rhesus haemolytic disease affected one in 20 babies with a 15% mortality rate. Those figures have now dropped to 2:1000 births with a less than 2% mortality rate (Bowman 1984; Terry 1990; Tovey 1990). The difficulty lies in the fact that HDN does still occur and continues to have potentially lethal affects on the fetus.

The effects of HDN were recognised in 1892 when Ballantyne referred to the symptoms of oedema, anaemia, hepatosplenomegaly and enlargement of the placenta as hydrops fetalis. In 1932 Darrow concluded that the formation of a maternal antibody against a component of fetal blood led to the symptoms of hydrops fetalis. The Rhesus antigen was discovered in 1940 by Landsteiner and Wiener, who found that 85% of caucasians carried the antigen. A year later, Levine et al confirmed that Rhesus sensitization did cause HDN and led to hydrops fetalis. The story was completed not long afterwards when Coombes developed an anti-human globulin test for the detection of incomplete antibodies (Bowman 1984; Dewhurst et al 1986; Fairweather 1989; Gravenhorst 1993; McDonald 1993).

The danger to the baby in a pregnancy affected by Rhesus incompatibility occurs because of mixing of the maternal and fetal circulations. Opportunities for this to happen are rare and in many cases no harm is done as the mother and fetus have compatible blood groups. In every pregnancy a small amount of fetal blood leaks into the maternal bloodstream. If this is Rh positive, approximately 5% of Rh negative primigravid women will develop a mild antibody response (Robertson 1986). But some women will go on to develop severe responses in the baby. The third stage of labour presents another opportunity. Rupture of the placental villi and connective tissue allows fetal red blood cells to escape into maternal circulation prior to constriction of the open maternal vessels (Dewhurst et al 1986; Gravenhorst 1993).

If the woman is Rhesus negative and the fetus is Rhesus positive, her bloodstream will identify the alien blood cells and respond by creating antibodies. Should this occur following the birth of the baby as the placenta is being delivered, no harm will come to the baby, but during the next pregnancy the antibodies will still be present in the maternal circulation and it is her blood which feeds the developing fetus. If the subsequent baby is also Rhesus positive, the antibodies will cross into the fetal circulation and begin to haemolyse the red blood cells; the process of haemolytic disease of the newborn begins and can result in the ultimate condition of hydrops fetalis as described above. With each successive pregnancy carrying a Rhesus positive fetus, larger amounts of antibody will be produced and the haemolytic disease in the baby will become more severe (Lenar and Harvey 1986).

Antepartum Haemorrhage

Antepartum haemorrhage is defined as bleeding from the genital tract after the fetus is viable (24 weeks gestation) (Sweet 1991b). There are three types of antepartum haemorrhage; the two main types are related to the placenta and can affect the viability of the fetus. The first is placental abruption and the second is placenta praevia. A third variety is bleeding from the cervix or vagina but this rarely compromises the fetus (Fraser and Watson 1993).

Placental abruption

Placental abruption occurs when a normally situated placenta separates from the uterine wall. The aetiology may be hard to identify, particularly as the diagnosis is often made in retrospect by the discovery of a retroplacental clot on the placenta (Fraser and Watson 1993). Abruption of the placenta has been associated with essential hypertension, pre-eclampsia, folic acid deficiency and trauma ((Naeye et al 1977; Sweet 1991a). The ensuing haemorrhage may be described as mild, moderate or severe depending on the actual blood loss, but the amount of bleeding does not represent a true guide as the abruption may be partially or wholly concealed. Warning signs may be evident in the form of bleeding, but this will depend on where the separation has occurred. If the edge of the placenta tears away from the uterine wall, the bleeding can escape and become evident, but if the edge of the placenta remains firmly adherent, the bleeding may not have the same opportunity and may present as 'spotting' or nothing at all. Dismissing a tiny amount of vaginal bleeding as insignificant could mean missing the potentially lethal abruption.

The perinatal mortality rate with confirmed placental abruption is high, often over 300 per 1000 births. Over half of these occur before the mother reaches hospital (Fraser and Watson 1993). When she does make it to hospital, the woman presents in severe pain and the abdomen is often tender and boardlike. There may be heavy vaginal bleeding as well. Following diagnosis of fetal death, the mode of delivery must be decided by the maternal clinical condition. Most obstetricians would favour a vaginal delivery unless contractions could not be stimulated or where clinical shock was uncontrollable (Fraser and Watson 1993).

Placenta praevia

Placenta praevia is defined as a placenta which is situated wholly or partially in the lower segment of the uterus. The incidence at term is 0.5–1% and the condition occurs more commonly in multigravid women (Sweet 1991b). There are assumed to be four classifications of placenta praevia. These are shown in Table 5.2.

The bleeding in placenta praevia occurs as the placenta separates from the wall of the uterus. As contractions commence, the lower uterine segment begins to stretch. The placenta is not capable of stretching and so the separation process begins. Warning signs may be evident with vaginal bleeding, usually in association with a contraction, and the woman may be admitted for investigation before the real danger occurs.

Owing to the presence of the placenta in the lower uterine segment, the presenting part may be high and possibly in the breech position. In addition, the fetal lie could be oblique. Abdominal palpation will reveal a soft, non-tender uterus. An ultrasound scan is often used to confirm the placental site and suspected diagnosis. The risk of inserting a finger through the soft, vascular placenta and causing a catastrophic haemorrhage is the reason why digital vaginal examination is contra-indicated in all cases of placenta praevia. However, the examination may be performed in the operating theatre, where it will be easy to proceed to caesarean section immediately if bleeding occurs (Sweet 1991b; Fraser and Watson 1993). The Confidential Enquiry into Maternal Deaths recommends the presence of a Consultant Obstetrician either to supervise or to perform this procedure

Table 5.2 Classification of placenta praevia (Sweet 1991b)

Type	Classification
Type I	Placenta mainly in the upper segment but encroaching on the lower segment
Type II	Placenta reaches to, but does not cover the internal os
Type III	Placenta covers the internal os when it is closed but not completely when it is dilated
Type IV	Placenta completely covers the internal os

(Department of Health 1994). Even in the situation where the baby has died *in utero*, a caesarean section may still be required if the placenta is obstructing the cervical os.

CAUSES OF STILLBIRTH: INFECTION

Pregnant women are subject to the same range of acute and chronic infections as non-pregnant women. The placenta acts as a barrier to protect the fetus from extrauterine infection, but certain microorganisms may cross the placenta to enter the fetal circulation. The damage caused by these organisms depends on the gestation at which the infection occurs and the vulnerability of the fetus at that time. The most common infections to affect the fetus are rubella, toxoplasmosis, cytomegalovirus, syphilis and group B streptococci.

Rubella

Rubella is a typical childhood illness which is mild in effect when contracted by non-pregnant women. If infection occurs during pregnancy, however, it can have devastating effects on the developing fetus. Selective immunisation programmes have been carried out in the United Kingdom, initially on schoolgirls aged 11–14 years but more recently extended to women of childbearing age who are seronegative (Wang and Smaill 1993). For some females the initial vaccine is sufficient to give lifetime protection, for others a booster is required.

If rubella is contracted during the pregnancy, the fetus develops a viraemia which inhibits cell division and causes defects in developing organs such as the brain, heart, ears and eyes. Infection during the first month of pregnancy is particularly dangerous and marginally less so for the following eight weeks (Miller et al 1982; Sweet 1991c). Wang and Smaill recommend voluntary termination of pregnancy following maternal infection during the first 16 weeks. If it is contracted during this period, counselling is difficult as fetal risks are not easy to determine (Wang and Smaill 1993).

Toxoplasmosis

Toxoplasmosis is an infection caused by the parasite *Toxoplasma gondii*. This microscopic single-cell organism is found in meat, in cat faeces, and in the soil where cats defecate (Parry 1993; Thow 1995). Cats are unique in being the only domestic animal in which

the reproductive cycle of *Toxoplasma gondii* takes place.
Toxoplasma gondii from cats can contaminate grazing land or grain
stores on farms. In this way animals and meat can become infected
(Thow 1995). Pregnant women are at risk through eating
contaminated meat, coming into contact with soil, at lambing time
if they live on a farm, and by handling cat litter (Ibarra 1992; Thow
1995).

Toxoplasmosis is generally asymptomatic in healthy adults
and individuals can only be affected once, so if a woman is immune
prior to pregnancy she will not transmit the organism to the baby
(Wang and Smaill 1993). When the infection occurs, the transfer
varies according to the gestation of the pregnancy. The
transmission rate in the first trimester is 17%, but this rises to
65% by the last month of pregnancy. Even though the rate
increases with the length of gestation, the effects on the fetus are
more severe the earlier the infection is transmitted. The baby may
develop severe symptoms including retinochoroiditis,
hydrocephalus and brain lesions. In early pregnancy, fetal death
and spontaneous abortion may occur. Prenatal screening by
amniocentesis or cordocentesis is possible if the woman is infected
(Parry 1993; Wang and Smaill 1993; Thow 1995).

Cytomegalovirus

Cytomegalovirus may be asymptomatic in the mother and cause
severe abnormalities in the developing fetus. The impact which the
virus can have is not restricted to the first trimester and a severe
infection can result in a stillbirth. Many pregnant women will
already be immune to the infection before conception; of the
remainder only a small proportion will lead to fetal disease (Sweet
1991c).

Syphilis

Syphilis during pregnancy allows the transfer of *Treponema
pallidum* from mother to baby, resulting in possible stillbirth
(Wang and Smaill 1993). Thankfully, the incidence of syphilis is
decreasing and evidence of the disease in babies is rare. If a
woman is infected, she may not experience symptoms and
serological screening is the only means of identifying whether the
fetus is at risk. Routine screening for this sexually transmitted
disease is performed at the onset of pregnancy; if a positive result
is found, treatment with antibiotics can cure the problem before
the baby is affected (Jewell 1990; Wang and Smaill 1993).

Group B streptococci

Infection with Group B streptococci is the most frequent cause of sepsis in the neonate. Babies of less than 2500 g are more prone to the infection, which has a rapid onset. The policy of administering prophylactic antibiotics to high-risk babies has proved less successful than was anticipated in overcoming the infection. Between 5% and 25% of pregnant women carry the organism in the genital tract and it appears that treatment during the antenatal period has only a transient effect on the vaginal flora (Anthony 1982). Treatment during the intrapartum period appears to have more effect but requires the identification of the woman at risk. Any woman presenting with prolonged rupture of the membranes, preterm labour or who exhibits signs of pyrexia should be investigated for infection (Wang and Smaill 1993).

Smoking

Cigarette smoking during pregnancy affects the ability of the fetus to grow. The damage is caused by the binding of carbon monoxide to the fetal haemoglobin, preventing the uptake of oxygen necessary for growth (Chappell and Lilley 1994). In excess of a hundred publications have noted that women who smoked during pregnancy had babies weighing an average of 200 g less than those of non-smoking women (Lumley and Astbury 1993). The difference was constant following adjustment for social class, maternal age, parity, education, height, weight, previous low-birthweight baby and alcohol consumption (Lumley and Astbury 1993; Chappell and Lilley 1994). The risk of a miscarriage or stillbirth is increased in smoking mothers (Chappell and Lilley 1994). Health education advice for pregnancy includes information on the influence of cigarette smoking, yet in 1990 28% of women continued to smoke during pregnancy (Stillbirth (Definition) Act 1992).

CAUSES OF STILLBIRTH: FETAL FACTORS

Fetal factors resulting in stillbirth are mainly congenital abnormalities. Those closely associated with fetal loss such as prematurity are generally caused by a maternal factor which influences fetal growth, gestational age or both. Placental abruption or premature rupture of the membranes lead to a preterm delivery of a small baby and to the potential for perinatal death. For this reason issues directly related to growth or prematurity will not be covered as a separate cause of death.

EXPERIENCING STILLBIRTH

The death of a baby before birth is a terrifying prospect for
pregnant women and their partners. The challenge to the medical
and midwifery staff is to ensure a standard of quality of care which
meets the individual needs of the couple. The doctor and the
midwife must be aware of the choices available and they must
consider the psychological as well as the physical implications of
the death. They must be able to acknowledge their own needs in
providing this care. A stillbirth may occur in advance of labour as
an intrauterine death or it may happen at the point of birth. The
level of shock and trauma caused by a stillbirth is equal regardless
of the circumstances, but differences in care may be needed
depending on when the stillbirth is identified.

In the event of a stillbirth during labour, the staff are
dealing with a couple suffering from immediate shock. The
midwives, obstetricians and paediatricians are also coming to
terms with the loss of the baby and have to be able to react
quickly. Where a baby is known to have died prior to labour, there
is more time to adjust, although for the parents the reality may not
be apparent until the moment of birth.

The declining number of stillbirths means that staff today are
less accustomed to dealing with this type of loss (Forrest 1982).
Over the last thirty years the incidence of intrapartum deaths has
decreased and now over 80% of deaths happen before the onset of
labour (MacFarlane et al 1986). The introduction of ultrasound
scanning has made the confirmation of fetal death much more
accurate. Keirse and Kanhai recommend that the diagnosis of fetal
death be made only when two experienced observers concur, either
after a sufficiently long and careful single ultrasound examination,
or after two separate examinations. Although this prolongs the
waiting period, they argue that women are prepared to wait if they
understand the reason for the delay (Keirse and Kanhai 1993).

A stillbirth may present in two ways: as an intrauterine
death or as an intrapartum death. The former is a death at some
time in the pregnancy after 24 weeks and before labour has
commenced. The latter happens during the actual labour.
Although there are many similarities in the care of both situations,
it is worth noting some of the differences which can present owing
to the initial circumstances.

Intrauterine Death

An intrauterine death is one which has occurred during the
pregnancy. There may be a variety of causes for the demise of the

baby and it may be days before the mother is aware of it. A lack of fetal movement tends to be the first indicator of a problem, raising the mother's fears and causing her to seek professional advice. Alternatively, she may discover the problem while attending for a routine investigation, such as an ultrasound scan. In this case the discovery is secondary to the reason for attending. The distress associated with the intrauterine death is quite intense. It includes feelings of guilt for not being more vigilant to the condition of the pregnancy and of guilt for not picking up early warning signs. This distress may be experienced by both the prospective parents and the health professionals involved (Stewart and Dent 1994). Guilt plays a large part in the emotional trauma following such an event and it is important that as much information as possible is gathered to determine the cause of death.

The decision about when to deliver the baby following a death *in utero* is often left to the woman. There is rarely a medical reason for inducing labour and time may be required for the woman and her partner to come to terms with the news before beginning labour. Alternatively, to continue the pregnancy in the knowledge that the outcome will be a dead baby may be worse for the couple and they may wish to be induced immediately (Kohn and Moffitt 1994).

Intrapartum Death

An intrapartum death is probably one of the worst possible scenarios for midwives and doctors to encounter. In this situation the death of the baby occurs during the actual labour. The prediction of fetal death may be possible from a number of clinical observations, such as severe fetal distress. With limited time to act, the priority is to ensure the safe delivery of the baby, perhaps at the expense of spending vital minutes explaining emergency procedures to the parents. It is extremely important that the staff take time to talk to the parents when the situation has calmed down.

On some occasions there are no warning signs and the death is discovered too late to attempt to save the baby. As with the intrauterine death, staff may be faced with a couple who have no indication that anything is wrong.

Hospital policy may dictate who is permitted to break the news of a baby's death. The parents will not be aware of protocol and may suspect that a problem has been identified. In these circumstances they are unlikely to want to wait for the designated person to arrive and may place the midwife, junior doctor or ultrasonographer in an awkward position by asking questions that the medical staff are forbidden to answer. Where a policy exists it must clearly take account of the members of staff who will be with the woman at the time a diagnosis of fetal death is made.

With a multiple pregnancy one of the babies may die; again this may be prior to labour or during the intrapartum phase. A decision may be made to induce the labour in order to protect the surviving baby or babies and the woman fully consulted about the process. At the time of delivery the staff are faced with the difficult situation of caring for a woman with at least one healthy baby and delivering a stillborn infant at the same time. It may be that the baby has been dead for some weeks, perhaps from the pre-viable stage but the actual gestation at the time of birth will dictate whether this baby is termed a stillbirth or a pre-viable fetus.

Labour Following an Intrauterine Death

When the diagnosis of intrauterine death has been confirmed, a decision must be made regarding labour and delivery. Spontaneous onset may take place and the midwives will monitor the progress as normal. Concern for fetal well-being during labour is replaced by the need to ensure that the birth is as easy as physically possible in the circumstances. The woman may be shocked to learn that she is still expected to experience labour and a request for caesarean section is not uncommon. Unfortunately, the potential risk to the maternal health from an operative procedure is sufficiently high to merit caution and it is rare for an obstetrician to consent to perform the operation. Experienced members of staff will have encountered this question on many previous occasions and should feel equipped to answer it in a sensitive manner, explaining all the reasons.

Time to adjust to the devastating news may be necessary before the couple can make any decisions about the birth. Staff need to ensure that they have privacy and the opportunity to talk and ask questions. It is important that the couple feel supported and that staff are not hurrying the process. The offer of a person of religious authority to help them at this time may be very welcome. An obvious difficulty is the inability of midwives or doctors to provide many answers at the beginning of the process. It may be too soon to discuss further than the actual immediacy of the loss, but the subject of postmortem examination can be sensitively raised as a means of attempting to find out as much as possible about the baby's death. There will be adequate time to follow these initial discussions in depth later.

Reassurance that adequate analgesia will be available is necessary and the presence of a familiar midwife will offer comfort. If the mother's health is uncompromised and the labour has not yet started, she may choose to go home and wait or she may decide on a particular time to be induced. The choice between active intervention and the expectant approach of allowing spontaneous labour is based on the emotional and psychological well-being of the woman. She is the best judge of the timing (Keirse and Kanhai 1993). An initial decision may be changed at any time and she should know how to communicate that change. She may already have a named midwife with whom she can maintain contact during this time; alternatively, she should know how to contact someone during this period. Communication with the delivery suite is important and the agreed time for induction must be confirmed with them. Once all the medical arrangements have been made, the woman may choose to return home and undergo any personal preparation she feels is necessary. Prior to her leaving the hospital the staff should ensure that she has a means to get home and is not stranded without cash or transport.

REFERENCES

Alberman E (1989) Perinatal mortality. In (A Turnbull & G Chamberlain, eds) *Obstetrics*, pp 117–122. Edinburgh, Churchill Livingstone.

Anthony BF (1982) Carriage of group B streptococci during pregnancy: A puzzler. *Journal of Infectious Diseases* **145**: 789–793.

Beischer NA & Mackay EV (1988) Perinatal mortality. In (NA Beischer & EV Mackay, eds) *Obstetrics and the Newborn*, pp 117–122. London, Baillière Tindall.

Bowman JM (1984) Rhesus haemolytic disease. In (NJ Wald, ed.) *Antenatal and Neonatal Screening*, pp 316–334. Oxford, Oxford University Press.

Chappell C & Lilley G (1994) Effects of smoking on the fetus and young children. *British Journal of Midwifery* **2**: 587–591.

Department of Health (1994) Antepartum and postpartum haemorrhage. In *Report on Confidential Enquiries into Maternal Deaths in the United Kingdom, 1988–1990*, pp 34–42. London, HMSO.

Dewhurst J, de Swiet M & Chamberlain GVP (1986) Rhesus incompatibility. In *Basic Science in Obstetrics and Gynaecology*, pp 203–205. Edinburgh, Churchill Livingstone.

Fairweather DVI (1989) Rhesus effect. In (A Turnbull & GVP Chamberlain, eds) *Obstetrics*, pp 503–513. Edinburgh, Churchill Livingstone.

Forrest GC (1982) Coping after stillbirth. In *Maternal and Child Health*, pp 394–398.

Fraser R & Watson R (1993) Bleeding during the latter half of pregnancy. In (I Chalmers, M Enkin and MJNC Keirse, eds) *Effective Care in Pregnancy and Childbirth*, pp 594–611. Oxford, Oxford University Press.

Gravenhorst JB (1993) Rhesus isoimmunization. In (I Chalmers, M Enkin & MJNC Keirse, eds) *Effective Care in Pregnancy and Childbirth*, pp 565–577. Oxford, Oxford University Press.

Hunter DJS (1994a) Diabetes in pregnancy. In (I Chalmers, M Ekin & MJNC Keirse, eds) *Effective Care in Pregnancy and Childbirth*, pp 578–593. Oxford, Oxford University Press.

Hunter DJS (1994b) Gestation diabetes. In (I Chalmers, M Enkin & MJNC Keirse, eds) *Effective Care in Pregnancy and Childbirth*, pp 403–410. Oxford, Oxford University Press.

Ibarra J (1992) Preventing toxoplasmosis. *Community Outlook* 2: 42–43.

Jewell D (1990) Prepregnancy and early pregnancy care. In (D Hall, ed.) *Antenatal Care*, pp 1–23. London, Baillière Tindall.

Keirse MJNC & Kanhai HHH (1993) Induction of labour after fetal death. In (I Chalmers, M Enkin & MJNC Keirse) *Effective Care in Pregnancy and Childbirth*, pp 1118–1126. Oxford Medical Publications, Oxford.

Kohn I & Moffitt PL (1994) Stillborn and newborn death. In *Pregnancy Loss*, pp 90–105. London, Hodder Headline.

Lenar CJH & Harvey D (1986) Rhesus incompatibility. In (CJH Kelnar & D Harvey, eds) *The Sick Newborn Baby*, pp 243–256. London, Baillière Tindall.

Lumley J & Astbury J (1993) Advice for pregnancy. In (I Chalmers, M Ekin & MJNC Keirse, eds) *Effective Care in Pregnancy and Childbirth*, pp 237–254. Oxford, Oxford University Press.

MacFarlane A, Cole S & Hey E (1986) Comparison of data from regional perinatal mortality surveys. *British Journal of Obstetrics and Gynaecology* **93**: 1224–1232.

Maresh M (1990) Medical complications in pregnancy. In (M. Hall, ed.) *Antenatal Care*, pp 129–147. London, Baillière Tindall.

McDonald M (1993) Rhesus incompatibility. *Nursing Times* **88**: 19.

Miller E, Cradock-Watson JE & Pollock TM (1982) Consequences of confirmed maternal rubella at successive stages of pregnancy. *Lancet* **ii**: 781–784.

Naeye RL, Harkes WL & Utts J (1977) Abruptio placentae and perinatal death: A prospective study. *American Journal of Obstetrics and Gynaecology* **128**: 701–704.

Parry V (1993) Routine tests. In *The Antenatal Testing Handbook*, pp 23–39. London, Pan Books.

Robertson NRC (1986) Pathological causes of jaundice. In *A Manual of Neonatal Intensive Care*, pp 211–219. London, Edward Arnold.

Stewart A & Dent A (1994) Death instead of life: At the time of birth or soon after. In (A Stewart & A Dent, eds) *At A Loss*, pp 51–74. London, Baillière Tindall.

Stillbirth (Definition) Act 1992. London, HMSO.

Sweet B (1991a) Bleeding in pregnancy. In (B Sweet, ed.) *Mayes' Midwifery*, 11th edn, pp 259–273. London, Baillière Tindall.

Sweet B (1991b) Associated conditions. In (B Sweet, ed.) *Mayes' Midwifery*, 11th edn, pp 289–303. London, Baillière Tindall.

Sweet B (1991c) Infections in the newborn. In (B Sweet, ed.) *Mayes' Midwifery*, 11th edn, pp 458–467. London, Baillière Tindall.

Terry PB (1990) Routine testing and prophylaxis. *Baillière's Clinical Obstetrics and Gynaecology* 4: no. 1. pp 25–43. London, Baillière Tindall.

Tew M (1995) Mortality of the child. In *Safer Childbirth*, pp 311–373. London, Chapman and Hall.

Thow S (1995) Maternal and congenital toxoplasmosis. *British Journal of Midwifery* 3: 129–132.

Tovey DLA (1990) Haemolytic disease of the newborn and its prevention. *British Medical Journal* 300: 313–316.

Wang E & Smaill F (1993) Infection in pregnancy. In (I Chalmers, M Enkin & MJNC Keirse, eds) *Effective Care in Pregnancy and Childbirth*, pp 534–564. Oxford, Oxford University Press.

Chapter Six

Postmortem Examination

"Why?"

The question on everybody's lips when a baby dies *in utero*, when a pregnancy ends in a miscarriage, when a fetal abnormality is diagnosed ... and for many more reasons. The answers are required immediately and are never enough. Doctors, nurses and midwives can be left feeling inadequate, unable to provide a solution which will reverse the diagnosis or alter the outcome. Hope for the future is required but not forthcoming. Time is required and assumptions are to be avoided. There may be a seemingly obvious reason why the baby has died, such as an umbilical cord around the neck; but this may mask the real cause of death in the form of a lethal, but unseen cardiac abnormality. The postmortem examination provides an opportunity to discover whether there is a reason for the baby's death.

The subject of postmortem examination is usually raised by the medical staff; on the whole doctors are more accustomed to discussing the subject than nursing or midwifery colleagues. More familiar with the procedure, the doctor can provide sufficient information and assistance for the couple to make their decision. The high percentage of postmortem examinations performed on babies are a credit to the sensitivity with which the subject is handled by obstetricians and midwives. If they are to serve their client well, the necessary information about the examination is required by midwives. Often, when the doctor has left the room, it is to the midwife that the couple turn and ask questions. The purpose of this chapter is to provide an insight into the procedure of the examination and to attempt to provide answers to some of the questions the midwife may be asked.

THE PATHOLOGIST

A relaxed everyday working relationship with neonatal and obstetric colleagues greatly improves the flow of clinical information.

(Chambers 1990)

The role of the histopathologist is to perform the postmortem examination. The pathology department may be familiar territory for midwives and nursing staff, but the mortuary is rarely visited and the role of the pathology staff may be poorly understood. An appreciation of the work involved in performing a postmortem examination may greatly assist communication with parents.

A specialist perinatal pathologist is employed within each Regional Health Authority. Their function is to provide additional support and advice to local pathology services. In cases of particularly rare fetal abnormalities it is necessary to have a resource person to rely on for confirmation and diagnosis of the suspected defects.

The audit of perinatal mortality should include regular meetings of the various professional groups including the pathology department. Depending on the different approaches within each hospital, this may provide the only opportunity to meet and discuss issues with the pathologist. Making a friend of your local pathologist may sound ridiculous, but the reality is that this person is responsible for much of the information which is passed to the mother after her baby has died.

CONSENT

Consent is generally obtained for all recognisable fetal remains to be examined. Obtaining consent for a postmortem examination can be one of the more difficult tasks in medicine. While the word 'childbirth' may be associated with pain, it is also synonymous with happiness. The prospect of consenting to a postmortem examination is something which few parents even consider during the pregnancy, thus making the reality of the situation even harder to accept. It is hardly surprising that the most common initial response is 'but he's suffered enough'. Or there may be sheer disbelief at the suggestion of cutting open their precious baby.

In situations of prenatal screening and diagnosis the postmortem examination may have been discussed in advance of the delivery. Although a decision may not have been reached, the first step in the process has been taken and this can only help the delivery team. Having trust in the staff who are caring for her will help the woman cope with the experience. The medical staff, appearing intermittently, do not always achieve the same degree of familiarity as the continual presence of the midwife. In situations of fetal loss this bond can be very strong and the client may depend heavily on the midwife's view. 'What would you do?' may be asked. It would be inappropriate for anyone other than the woman and her partner to take responsibility for this decision. Enabling their client to make an informed choice is the direction in which staff should be aiming.

POSTMORTEM
EXAMINATION
– The Pathologist
– Consent
– Time
– Changing Decision
– P.M. Objections

TIME

Deciding for or against a postmortem may take considerable time for the woman. If she has a partner, then two people have to be happy with the decision reached, and this may add extra trauma to their grief if there is disagreement.

The relationship between the midwife and the woman may have started in the antenatal period, and if continuity can be provided in labour the trust tends to strengthen and grow. Questions which may be difficult to ask can be broached to a familiar person and the, sometimes hidden, message revealed to the midwife who knows her client well.

CHANGING THE DECISION

Allowing the woman and her partner sufficient time to reach a decision is important. The need to complete the paperwork before discharge can be an overlooked burden to the parents; it should not matter if they wish to have more time to think. The midwife will have encouraged them to discuss the matter together and ask as many questions as necessary. The doctor or midwife may have a personal view on the decision but the baby does not belong to them. It is both unfair and unwise for the health professional to attempt to change the couple's mind in one direction or another. The parents are the people who have to live with their choice for the rest of their lives. If they choose to change their minds at any time, they should know who to contact. For this reason it is beneficial to inform the parents of the time that the examination will take place.

OBJECTION TO POSTMORTEM

In certain situations consent may be refused because of religious or cultural beliefs. Alternatively, the consent may be given, but with certain stipulations to ensure that any religious requirements are met (Hanid 1980). Strong negative feelings may exist about the benefits of performing the examination. Death is usually associated with pain and suffering, and for many people it is hard to imagine that a postmortem will not cause pain. Parents of a dead baby may find the prospect of 'inflicting' pain on their innocent child too upsetting even to contemplate. There may also be a real fear of how the baby will look following the examination.

THE POSTMORTEM EXAMINATION PROCEDURE

The postmortem examination may be performed in the hospital where the baby has been born. Alternatively the body may be transferred to a specialist pathologist, usually at a nearby teaching hospital. Perinatal postmortem examination is an integral supplement to prenatal diagnosis and as a result the demand for specialist pathology is increasing. The specialist perinatal pathologist will have greater experience of the rare congenital abnormalities which are not seen frequently in district hospitals.

Transport

Consideration must be given to the condition of the baby while on the ward area. The baby needs to be suitably cared for and a refrigerator may be sufficient for a short period of time. Much depends on the wishes of the mother at this time, but guidance from the staff will help her to appreciate the need to care for the baby properly. Handing the baby over to staff for transfer to the mortuary may be particularly difficult for the mother; consideration of her needs at this time should avoid the process being more painful than necessary. Reassurance about where the baby is being taken and how long it will be before they can see him or her again must be given (Henley and Kohner 1991).

   If transfer to another pathology department is required, guidelines must be in place to ensure this is done appropriately. Mistakes can occur and can lead to unnecessary distress for the mother and unwanted publicity for the hospital. Indeed, in 1995, *The Guardian* newspaper reported how a body had been transported to another hospital in a cardboard box. The box had got wet but the hospital reported that the body was inside a sealed plastic container (*Guardian* 1995). For transfers of any distance, a funeral director or hospital transport should be used. All relevant maternal and obstetric details should accompany the body.

   Before being placed in the container for transfer the baby must be clearly identified in the same manner as a live birth. The mother may have chosen to dress her baby while he or she was with her on the ward; while this is not to be deterred, clothes and blankets do speed up the process of autolysis and the pathologist may ask for them to be removed before the baby leaves the ward.

The midwife will be able to reassure the mother than the baby can be dressed again for the funeral if she chooses.

Remembering to save the placenta for histological examination can be a problem as the trend is to dispose of all placentae and there are many other practical issues to consider. But the placenta may provide clues to the cause of death and can be valuable if consent for postmortem is not granted.

The postmortem consent form should accompany the body. It can be very distressing for the doctor who sees the woman for her follow-up appointment to have to admit that the baby was released for burial before the postmortem was performed as the consent form had got lost. Having agonised over the decision she is unlikely to take this information well.

The Examination

Guidelines for perinatal postmortem examination were drawn up by the Confidential Enquiry into Stillbirths and Deaths in Infancy (CESDI) and approved by the Royal College of Pathologists in May 1993. The guidelines were considered to be the minimum requirements and advocated the use of individual clinical judgement to conduct specialist investigations as indicated by the case of family history (Department of Health 1993a; Department of Health 1993b).

Histological examination of the various organs of the body is critical. The results may take days or weeks to be produced and affect the availability of the final report in the first days following the postmortem.

Sites for incision on the body have been modified in recent years, coinciding with the increase in requests to view the baby after the procedure. The majority of pathologists will access the cranial area from an arc across the skull, an 'Alice band' line. To gain entry to the organs of the trunk a Y-shaped incision may be used; alternatively a vertical cut is made from neck to trunk.

Repairing the Body

Repair of the body may be influenced by the knowledge that the family may wish to hold the baby (Knowles 1994). Repair also depends on the condition and gestational age of the baby. A very small or macerated baby can be difficult to reconstruct. The person responsible for the repair is usually the mortuary attendant or technician, who will endeavour to create the right appearance. Replacement of major organs to their original position is not always done and gauze or cotton wool may be used to pad out the cranial area. When the family do choose to hold the baby again the lightness of the head may cause surprise. Having observed families in rural Australia, where he is part of a perinatal loss support team, Knowles acknowledges that this has changed his practice. He has refined his technique to ensure that organs are replaced appropriately and a contract is made with the mother about the extent of her consent to the procedure (Knowles 1994). In some instances the postmortem form includes information that certain organs may be retained; parents are not always clear about this and may be distressed to discover too late that it has happened.

Superglue or dental floss may be used to reappose the skin edges in place of suture material. While they are equally effective, the difference is made in the invisible nature of the repair. Despite the efforts made to return the baby to a reasonable condition, staff would be advised to encourage the taking of photographs before the postmortem examination rather than afterwards.

Releasing the Body for Disposal

The baby will be available for burial or cremation as soon as the postmortem has been completed. By this time the mother may have decided on the form of burial or cremation and communicated with a funeral director who will contact the hospital.

Results

Results from the postmortem examination may take up to six weeks to be available. An appointment with the Consultant Obstetrician or Paediatrician should be given for the six-week limit. The interval will ensure that all results have been returned. A joint clinic may be held with the obstetric and paediatric consultants. In the majority of cases of perinatal loss the midwife will have been the main provider of care and, although her professional responsibility to the woman is over by this time, the midwife's attending the appointment can be beneficial for all parties, especially if the woman has not met the consultant before. The appointment needs to allow time for questions and repetition of previously mentioned facts which have not been understood properly. Account should be taken of the needs of women whose first language is not English, to enable them to be fully informed about their care (Department of Health 1993a).

The postmortem examination may provide a specific cause of death, and it can correct clinical impressions and identify genetic factors requiring further assessment and counselling (Meier et al 1986). Alternatively, the examination may not reveal an apparent cause of death, a very positive fact for future pregnancies. How this positive news is interpreted by the parents may depend on the way it is relayed to them. If the attitude is apologetic in nature then they may be disappointed with the outcome, possibly angry that they have 'put their baby through the process' without finding any answers. An alternative attitude may help them to understand that an unknown cause of death will have ruled out most of the major abnormalities and congenital problems which can be identified at postmortem examination. For this reason they can embark on future pregnancies with less anxiety and doubt about the outcome.

Conclusion

Perinatal postmortem examination is recommended in all cases of fetal death. A postmortem following a therapeutic termination of pregnancy will, it is hoped, confirm the diagnosis as being correct. The procedure may also detect additional, significant abnormalities. The responsibility for the postmortem examination rests with the pathologist. The midwife and doctor who address the issue with the mother and her partner have a responsibility to provide every opportunity for the cause of death to be determined. Those purchasing maternity services have a responsibility to ensure that the option of a postmortem examination is given due attention and importance in the negotiating of contracts and is clear in service specifications for the consumers they represent. The providers have a responsibility to offer the service to a high standard of quality and in line with the recommendations of the Royal College of Pathologists and the guidelines of the Confidential Enquiry into Stillbirths and Deaths in Infancy.

REFERENCES

Chambers HM (1990) The perinatal autopsy. *Medical Journal of Australia* **153**: 578–579.

Department of Health (1993a) Making best use of the service. In *Changing Childbirth*, pp 55–56. London, HMSO.

Department of Health (1993b) *The Confidential Enquiry into Stillbirths and Deaths in Infancy: Report March 1992–July 1993*. London, HMSO.

Guardian (1995) 'Caring Staff' Praised after Hospital sent Body in Parcel, 10 Feb.

Hanid TK (1980) Islam and postmortem examination. *The Journal of Child and Maternal Health*. Mar.: 95.

Henley A & Kohner N (1991) The postmortem laboratory investigations. In *Guidelines for Professionals*, pp 45–48. London, SANDS.

Knowles S (1994) A passage through grief: The Western Australia Rural Pregnancy Loss Team. *British Medical Journal* **309**: 1705–1708.

Meier PR, Manchester DK, Shikes RH, Clewell WH & Stewart M (1986) Perinatal autopsy: Its clinical value. *Obstetrics and Gynaecology* **67**: 349–351.

Chapter Seven

Religious Aspects

The impact of religion on people's lives varies enormously, from an annual Christmas visit to Midnight Service to a total commitment to the teachings of the particular faith. To complicate matters further, religious faith may alter at different times and be significantly influenced by certain life events. In grief a lapsed faith may be rekindled or a deep belief lost. Individuals respond in their own unique ways. Often it is hard for family or friends to understand what is happening as they may only have a 'snapshot' view of the illness or event which has occurred and lack an understanding of some underlying issues. The health professional has to adapt to the different religions of his or her clients and their particular needs in relation to these.

Religion and culture are inextricably linked and the purchasing authority has to recognise this when negotiating contracts for care. In large cities where populations may be divided into particular religious groups the serving hospital may adapt to provide accordingly. For example, the trust may provide a Muslim chaplain if there is a large Muslim community within the area. The variants of care pertinent to each religion require some consideration in order for staff to avoid causing offence. There is also the need to consider the religious beliefs of the doctors, nurses, midwives and support staff.

The purpose of this chapter is to observe the more commonly found religions and their particular beliefs in relation to the death of a baby before birth. This may be a difficult task owing to the wide range of religions in Britain today and the individual interpretation placed upon many of them. For some religious groups the newborn baby has no claim on the rituals of death which apply to older children or adults. There is a limited supply of written information available and I am grateful to those religious groups who offered verbal support, invited me to their meetings and were willing to discuss the subject and to speak for a wider membership. The overwhelming message was that each mother is an individual and, despite what it may say on her casenotes about religion, the best approach is to ask her.

THE HOSPITAL CHAPLAIN

Hospitals have been required to appoint chaplains from the main denominations since 1949. The responsibility of the chaplain is to minister to the needs of the patients and staff as required. If unable to meet the individual's needs the chaplain may seek assistance from other religious persons (Hospital Chaplaincies Council 1993).

In the majority of NHS Trust hospitals a chapel is provided. The chapel is available to all staff, visitors and patients throughout the day and may also be used for Christian services on a regular or occasional basis. Arrangements for other denominations will depend on the individual hospital.

The number of chaplains attached to a hospital may vary. Contact and close liaison with other clergy is essential. Religious support may be required at any time of the day or night and staff should know how to contact the chaplain if necessary. The need to see or talk to the chaplain may be identified by the nursing, midwifery or medical staff, who can act as advocate for the client. Alternatively, the client or her relatives or friends may make the request. For the chaplain, the call to a bedside can present difficulties, especially if there is a lack of information or a language barrier. Staff can do a lot to assist the chaplain by providing the relevant history. Interpreters may be requested to assist with a visit to a non-English-speaking woman. In some instances an interpreter may not be available or appropriate and the chaplain must decide how to proceed. It may be that non-verbal communication can provide all the support and comfort needed.

With specific regard to the area of perinatal loss, staff may have worked at the hospital for a long time and had regular contact with the chaplain. They need to be aware of changes to the role and new appointments, say an inexperienced chaplain who has never come across a dead baby before. If the dead baby is still in the room, the chaplain should be informed before entering so that he or she is prepared. The approach may be that the midwife caring for the woman introduces the chaplain to the client and the baby at the same time. The chaplain will have a wider remit than the immediately bereaved and may be required to support the family and friends who are present. Recognition should be given to the grief the family are exposed to, regardless of the gestational age at which the baby has died.

A basic understanding of the language of perinatal loss and the particular guidelines and protocols provided by the hospital is necessary. In order to meet the pastoral needs of a transient congregation the chaplain must appreciate the process of dying within the hospital environment. Death is an integral part of hospitals and the chaplain is regularly involved. The chaplain can be a key person involved in drawing up guidelines for care on both the maternity unit and the gynaecology ward (Smith 1993). The disposal arrangements following the death of a fetus or baby are areas which the chaplain should be familiar with. At the mother's request the chaplain may be the liaison person for the funeral.

RELIGIONS AND CULTURES

From long-established immigrant communities to recently arrived ethnic groups, the British Isles are a kaleidoscope of cosmopolitan cultures and religious observations. Hospital staff are constantly required to provide holistic care to their patients/clients and may struggle to overcome the confusion inspired by some of the religions practised in Britain today (Sampson 1982; Lothian Racial Equality Council 1992; Hospital Chaplaincies Council 1993).

A culture may be defined as the way of living adopted by the people in a particular group. The culture develops in response to the needs of the individuals and may change to resolve issues which arise. When group members move they take the culture with them, to adhere to or adapt to the new surroundings (Lothian Racial Equality Council 1992).

Staff will also have their own religious beliefs and customs. It is important that they do not slip into the trap of offering advice to the woman based on their own religious position (Stewart and Dent 1994). Midwives, doctors and nursing staff have a responsibility to the women in their care to understand the religions and ethnic groups to which they belong (Mander 1994). Rituals may be cathartic, allowing the opportunity to grieve in public. Attendance at a funeral ceremony can signify the reality of the death. It is not unusual for lapsed practitioners to rediscover a belief in their faith at times of terminal illness or death (Kohn and Moffitt 1994).

Termination of pregnancy raises concerns for many religions who do not believe that there is ever a reason to do so. For a woman whose religion forbids termination under any circumstances there are additional worries about going against her Church's wishes and the guilt which may be associated with this. Even when a religion does not specifically reject termination it can be difficult to make a decision. Help in the form of guidance and advice from a clerical/religious leader is the best solution; in this way the individual circumstances can be discussed. The view may be unchanged but the woman may have greater peace with herself about making her choice.

Buddhism

Buddhism began in Nepal, north of the Himalayas in Northern
India in the sixth century BC. The name Buddha means the
Enlightened. It was a name bestowed upon a young Indian,
Siddhattha who lived in the region (Hennells 1984). Tradition tells
of the experiences of Siddhattha leading to his enlightenment at
Bodhaya and his subsequent journeyings in northern India as one
of the wandering ascetic philosophers of the day. The faith of
Buddhism centres around the Buddha, who is revered as a way of
life rather than as a god (Green 1994).

Followers do not worship Buddha as he is not revered as a
god. Instead they follow Buddhism as a tradition of thought and
practice. The Buddha's way was set out in three basic beliefs: *Sila*
(morality), *Samadhi* (meditation) and *Panna* (wisdom). The
disciples attracted to Buddhism formed a community who follow a
Vinaya or discipline. After his death the Buddha's teachings
continued to be used and schools emerged. Lay followers of
Buddhism concentrate on the pursuit of morality and the giving of
alms. They also recognise special days in the Buddhist calendar
and actively participate in a number of festivals in honour of
Buddha. There are approximately 20,000 Buddhists in Britain.

Therapeutic termination of pregnancy

Buddhists do not accept termination of pregnancy.

Death

One of the first things which must be done when a Buddhist dies is
to inform a Buddhist monk, preferably one from the same school of
Buddhism as the deceased (there are three schools in Britain)
(Green 1994). When a baby dies, the midwife or the parents should
contact a monk or minister from the same school as the parents.

It is acceptable to follow the normal practice for the dead
when caring for a Buddhist baby.

Postmortem

A postmortem examination is acceptable within the Buddhist
religion (Green 1994).

Funerals

In a country where Buddhism is the main religion, the deceased
are placed on a platform in a central area of the town or village.
Death is not a closed, private affair and friends are encouraged to
pay their respects in public. Meditation is encouraged to
contemplate and relinquish the dead.

A Buddhist follower believes that, as the body is made up of elements such as minerals and plants which belong to the earth, then the body should be returned to the earth. Cremation is the usual form of disposal of the body. If ashes are available, they can be returned to the earth in a graceful way. A tree is planted where the remains have been left. The tree symbolises the rebirth and the completion of the cycle. Readings at the ceremony vary according to the Buddhist school and may include mantras for compassion and purification of the dead (Dhammarati 1989; Sucitto 1989; Green 1994).

For a certain number of days following the death there may be chanting. The purpose of this is to remember the deceased as a human being. After a period of one hundred days a second ceremony is held on a smaller scale. At this ceremony the deceased is commemorated by the burning of a photograph of the individual. In this way total relinquishing of the dead can occur. At each of these events important emphasis is placed on grief and mourning. In general the process of death is recognised as a significant event and there is a general acceptance that mourning will take a long time to complete.

Christianity

The Anglican church

Almost one-third of the world's population profess some form of Christianity (Green 1994; Hennells 1984). Christianity spread following the ministry of Jesus Christ and has survived many reformations and divisions. By the sixteenth century, reformation and counter-reformation had split the Western church into two broad groups: Roman Catholicism and Protestantism. The latter group split further, creating many new churches and sects (Hennells 1984). The Anglican church is the acknowledged Church of England; its dogma is also common in the Church of Wales, the Church of Ireland and the Episcopalian Church in Scotland. One over-riding concept is that of a single God who reveals Himself as the Father, the Son and the Holy Spirit (Green 1994). Approximately 57% of British people declare themselves to be followers of the Anglican religion (Green 1994).

Baptism

Anglicans believe that baptism into the faith will lead to a share in Christ's resurrection and eternal life. Baptism is associated with the naming of the baby or child. If the child is born dead the ritual of baptism may be omitted and the parents could be concerned that the baby will be excluded from entering the Kingdom of God.

Reassurance and advice may be sought from the hospital chaplain and a special blessing may be performed.

If there are signs of life present at the delivery, the parents may request that an immediate baptism be performed. In an emergency of this nature it is acceptable for a member of staff who is of the same faith to stand in for the priest. A ceremony of baptism may not be performed on a baby who is born dead; instead a blessing is said and the name given (Green 1994).

Postmortem

There are no religious objections to a postmortem examination.

Funerals

A baby of the Anglican faith may be buried or cremated.

The Roman Catholic church

The Roman Catholic faith is a form of Christianity. The major difference between it and other Christian denominations is that it accepts the supremacy of the Bishop of Rome (the Pope) as absolute. The word 'catholic' is from the Greek meaning 'general' or 'universal'. Roman Catholics make up the majority of the world's Christian religious believers.

Baptism

Baptism is extremely important to the Catholic religion and parents may request the presence of a priest for the birth of the baby. A blessing may be performed if signs of life are not present.

Termination of pregnancy

Termination of pregnancy for any reason is forbidden in the teaching of the Roman Catholic Church. Procreation of life is considered sacred and interference with that process is not acceptable in any form.

Postmortem examination

Consent to postmortem examination may be given by the parents without objection.

Funerals

Burial or cremation are both acceptable practices.

Free churches

In addition to the Anglican and Roman Catholic faiths there are many denominations within the free church. The churches which make up the free churches originated in the Reformation. The following list are those given by Sampson as components of the Free Church Federal Council which was founded in 1940:

- The Baptist Union of Great Britain and Ireland
- The Churches of Christ
- The Congregational Foundation
- The Countess of Huntingdon's Connexion
- The Independent Methodist Churches
- The Methodist Church
- The Moravian Church
- The Presbyterian Church of Wales
- The Salvation Army
- The Union of Welsh Independents
- The United Reformed Church
- The Wesleyan Reform Union (Sampson 1982)

Other faiths come under the care of the free church chaplain within the hospital. The chaplain will always know how to contact an appropriate religious person. There are many other sects who are not included in the Council such as the Plymouth Brethren or the Church of Scotland and the Quakers.

Although some of the sects do have a specific view about issues such as termination of pregnancy, the tendency appears to be to encourage individual choice. For all aspects of perinatal loss the hospital chaplain will be able to advise about who to contact. The decision on baptism, burial and postmortem examination can be left to the conscience of the individual but they may seek guidance from a member of their own faith.

Baptism

The view of many of the groups is that baptism may not be essential; no alternative is required (Green 1994).

Postmortem examination

Religious groups within the free churches do not have objections to postmortem examination.

Funerals

Burial and cremation are equally acceptable.

Chinese Religions

The majority of Chinese people follow three religious beliefs, taking ideas and practices from each. The three great traditions are those of Confucianism, Taoism and Buddhism (Hennells 1984).

Confucius is probably the best-known thinker in Chinese history. Travelling through his native land he attempted to advise different federal rulers and gained a small following of disciples. The term 'Taoism' means Teachings of the Way and is used to refer to followers seeking access to the Tao as the supreme reality and consequent immortality. There are various legends about the entry of Buddhism into China at very early dates. According to Hennells the framework for Chinese public life and for family and social values is based on the teachings of Confucius; the Taoist influence results in the quest for immortality, and Buddhism represents the importance of abstinence and restraint as demonstrated by the Buddhist monks (Hennells 1984).

Termination of pregnancy

The termination of pregnancy for fetal abnormality is not objected to in any of the Chinese religions.

Postmortem

There are no formal objections to a postmortem examination.

Funerals

In accordance with the differing aspects of the Chinese religions there are many influences on the funeral process. Much may depend on the financial position of the family and the traditional aspects of their beliefs.

Hinduism

The range of beliefs and practices of Hindus is wide and varied. The term Hindu was first used by invading Muslims to describe the inhabitants of the 'land beyond the Indus river' (Hennells, 1984). Hindus are mainly found in the Indian continent but are also apparent in countries to which Indians have migrated. The caste system within Indian culture leads to a variety of interpretations of the rituals and laws of the religion.

The Hindu religion centres around a Guru who can be worshipped and understood in many forms. Hindus believe in reincarnation and think that the behaviour of the person in the present life influences the caste and status of the individual when he or she returns in the next. In this way each person is responsible for their own future (Green 1994).

Hindu women will generally prefer female nurses, doctors and midwives. In the event of a death a Hindu priest may be needed to support the parents and immediate family.

Following the birth of a baby the Hindu woman is considered to be at her weakest and the female members of the family may attend to her at home. She may be required to conform to the forty-day lying in period which is used to safeguard against infection and backache. In the case of a dead baby the woman may still adhere to this advice and support.

Termination of pregnancy

Consent to terminate a pregnancy is not usually granted by the parents, even in the event of a diagnosed abnormality. Difficulties may arise when there is known to be a consanguineous marriage which has resulted in a pregnancy with a diagnosed abnormality. The parents may speak limited English, particularly the woman, and an interpreter may be required to ensure that the parents have a full understanding.

In the event of a mother becoming seriously ill during the pregnancy, where terminating the pregnancy would be required, such as with severe pre-eclampsia, the mother's life takes precedence over the unborn baby and in this case a termination would be acceptable.

Postmortem examination

Although the general impression may be of condemnation of a postmortem, nothing in the Hindu religion specifically prohibits the procedure.

Funerals

All adult Hindus are cremated, but children and babies may be buried. The disposal of the body should ideally take place within 24 hours.

Islam

Islam is traditionally regarded as the final revelation of God's (Allah's) wishes to the Prophet Mohammed. The word 'Islam' means 'submission to God' and is interpreted as an unconditional surrender (Hennells 1984). From the early beginnings in western Arabia, Islam has spread worldwide: the number of followers is currently estimated at 800 million (Hennells 1984; Green 1994). Although scattered globally, the centre of the Islamic faith remains in the Arabic area. Mecca, by the Red Sea is a place of pilgrimage which all Muslim people aspire to visit in their lifetime.

Muslims regard the body as sacred. As a consequence, a Muslim woman may request female doctors, nurses and midwives. Internal vaginal examinations may be refused during labour.

Termination of pregnancy

In general the pregnancy may be terminated if the mother's health is thought to be in danger.

Postmortem examination

As the body is considered to belong to Allah, consent for postmortem examination is likely to be refused.

Funerals

Following death the body must be cared for by a Muslim. If the baby is handled by anyone other than a Muslim, disposable gloves should be worn. Burial within 24 hours is preferred. Immediately following the death the body should be laid straight and the head turned to the right, positioned so that the body is facing Mecca (in Great Britain this is to the South East). The eyes and mouth should be closed and the body washed twice, concentrating on the usual ablutions first. Soap, water and possibly disinfectant should be used. A sheet should be used to cover the baby completely. When the baby has been cleaned according to Muslim custom, a musk perfume may be applied before the body is wrapped in a clean white sheet.

In the case of a stillbirth the usual funeral prayer is omitted. It would not be usual for the body of a Muslim to be placed in a wooden coffin. According to Islamic law the area above the burial site must be slightly raised and the body buried, facing Mecca, in an unmarked grave. In Great Britain a professional funeral director should be engaged to handle the body and prepare the funeral. Muslims must always be buried, never cremated. The burial should not be delayed unnecessarily. In some instances the family may wish to take the body home to their native country for burial. The funeral director can help to arrange this. After the burial the family will usually attend the grave for forty days to say daily prayers for the deceased.

Jehovah's Witnesses

The Jehovah's Witness movement was founded by Charles Taze Russell in America in the nineteenth century. Followers attempt to live their lives in accordance with the commands of God in the Old and the New Testaments. The Bible is interpreted literally and there is a belief that the Kingdom of God will be experienced on earth and that followers will be resurrected following their death (Green 1994). Followers are committed to spreading the word and there are no separate clergy. Jehovah's Witnesses live plainly and reject stimulants and blood transfusions. Blood is considered to be the 'soul of the flesh' and must not be taken into the body in any form, including blood products such as plasma, packed cells and platelets. In the event of a baby requiring a blood transfusion, possibly an intrauterine infusion for severe rhesus incompatibility, the parents will most likely refuse.

Baptism

Baptism of a Jehovah's Witness does not generally occur before the age of twelve. Children under that age are protected by their parents and would not require baptism if their life was in danger. Therefore it is not necessary to baptise a baby at the time of birth or to perform a ceremony of blessing.

Postmortem examination

When alive the body is sacred to the Jehovah's Witness, but there is no objection to a postmortem examination. The decision would be left to the parents of the individual baby.

Funerals

Burial and cremation are acceptable for babies. Each service is individually prepared. The ceremony normally takes place at the local 'Kingdom Hall', which is the meeting place of the followers.

Judaism

Judaism is the religion of the Jewish people. Jewish religion and culture are woven closely together and the name Jew has been recognisable since the sixth century BC. Belief is in one God who judges the actions of man, who rewards and punishes according to how a person lives their life and who will send a Messiah to usher in the redemption. The Torah contains the Ten Commandments which God gave to Moses and which determine Jewish values (Hennells 1984).

The Sabbath is the Jewish holy day of obligation which commences at sunset of Friday afternoon and ends with the first sighting of three stars on Saturday night. As the Sabbath ends, a candle is lit and a blessing is said for the coming week. If an Orthodox Jew is in hospital she may still wish to observe the Sabbath and would appreciate the assistance of staff in conforming to the requirements.

There are different types of Judaism and a variety of interpretations of the teachings and observance of the religion.

Sefardim

The majority of Jews found in Islamic countries are Sephardic. Originally of Spanish origin, they left Spain and Portugal in the fifteenth century and settled in North America, the Far East and Northern Europe. More than half the population of Israel consists of Sephardi Jews. The Sephardi Jew differs from the Ashkenazi Jew in cultural habits and ritual ways. For the most part, cultural differences have resulted because exiled Jews settling in other countries have adapted the religion to incorporate some of the local traditions of their new homelands.

Ashkenazim

The term 'Ashkenazi' originally meant 'German' and was applied to Jews of central and eastern Europe. Ashkenazi Jews split from the Sephardi Jews (of Spanish or Portuguese descent) in the Middle Ages and developed their own customs and traditions of interpreting the Talmud, a collection of ancient writings on Jewish civil and ceremonial law and tradition. The pronunciation of Hebrew changed and some words were adopted into the new language of Yiddish, a language based on an old German dialect. Both Ashkenazi and Sephardi Jews remain true to the basic Jewish practice and theology.

Chasidism or Hasidism

Israel Baal Shem Tov founded Chasidism in the eighteenth century. Early centres were in the Ukraine and Southern Poland but Chasidism has now spread throughout Europe. The teaching of Chasidism focuses on the importance of serving God in day-to-day activities, especially in times of joy. This Jewish sect has turned its back on many of the ritual Jewish laws and is often criticised by the Jews of a more orthodox faith.

Reform Judaism

The traditional beliefs and practices of Judaism were challenged in the nineteenth century and Reform Judaism began as a response to this. From the beginning, the movement in Europe has been divided between radicals and moderates. This is often reflected in the approach to teachings of the faith and should be considered when treating a Reform Jew.

In Britain Reform Judaism has remained more true to the traditional line of teaching than the radical approach taken in North America.

Termination of pregnancy

The preservation of life is an important guiding principle in Judaism. The acceptance of termination of pregnancy may only be possible if the mother's life is in danger.

Postmortem examination

Postmortem examination is not generally accepted. In each situation the parents should be given the opportunity to discuss their fears or concerns.

Funerals

The death of a baby at the time of birth is no different in principle from other deaths. The Jewish burial authorities should be informed within 24 hours of the death and burial should take place as soon as possible. Funerals do not take place on the Sabbath.

The baby should be left in a separate room, but not in a mortuary if it is consecrated for Christian purposes. The baby's arms should be laid straight at the sides of the body and the eyes and mouth closed. Hospital staff may assist with these preparations but anything extra should be left to the Jewish authorities. The nursing and midwifery staff will be asked to show their respect to the baby by doing nothing further to him or her. The room should not contain a crucifix or other symbol of Christian faith. If there is no alternative a cloth should be used to cover the Christian symbols (Jacobs 1994).

If the death of the baby has occurred on the Sabbath or on a Jewish festival, nothing can be done to the body until the end of the day. During these events the rabbi will not answer his telephone, although there is no objection to somebody visiting him personally to inform him. For the family or relatives to make the funeral arrangements, they will have to contact the Burial Authority of their own synagogue. They may also be advised to inform the local Synagogue Office (Office of the Chief Rabbi 1994).

In the event of a perinatal death there is no obligation of *Keriah* (i.e. the tearing of the clothes). Nor is it necessary to have a *Minyan* (ten men) at the service as the *Kaddish* prayer is not obligatory. *Kaddish* is considered to apply to those who have 'a presumption of life'. This is not felt to occur before the first thirty days of life (Office of the Chief Rabbi 1994). Prayers recited include the memorial prayer and the prayer for the bereaved with some omissions from the text. The minister is left to choose the psalms and, although a eulogy for the departed is not possible, words of comfort for the parents are generally offered. The naming of the baby should take place before the burial to ensure that no life is anonymous. In the case of a male infant the *Brit* (circumcision) is formally performed by the Burial Authority at the time the burial preparations are made. Only after the *Brit* is the name chosen. For a female infant the name is chosen before the funeral service.

The parents may decide for themselves whether to attend the funeral. The length of time for mourning is determined by Biblical law relating to the redemption of the firstborn. In the case of a stillborn baby the usual period of mourning is not observed as the life was less than thirty days.

A tombstone may be erected on the grave and inscribed with the baby's name. Marking the anniversary of the death may include the lighting of the Yahrzeit candle. The Synagogue Office may agree to an *Aliyah* (call-up) to the Torah.

Mormons

The Mormon Church is correctly known as the Church of Jesus Christ of Latter-Day Saints and was founded in the United States by Joseph Smith in the nineteenth century. Joseph Smith claimed to translate the Book of Mormon, a supplement to the Old and New Testaments of the Bible. There is a belief in both pre-existence and resurrection. The first is a spirit world prior to birth on earth, of which the living have no memory. Following death it is believed that the spirit and the body are reunited and resurrection takes place. As with the Hindu approach to resurrection, the Mormon faith believes that a person's behaviour in the present life determines their fortune in the next.

Great emphasis is placed on the family. A posthumous contract for the baptism of the deceased may be undertaken by the living to ensure that all loved ones are united in faith. Death is considered to be a temporary separation (Green 1994).

Baptism

Children are not baptised until the age of eight, so it is not imperative to arrange baptism or a blessing following a stillbirth.

Postmortem examination

There is no religious objection to a postmortem examination.

Funerals

Burial of the baby would be preferred to cremation but the doctrine of the Church is not dictate absolute. The service will be held at the Church Meeting House.

Rastafarianism

The Rastafarian Movement began in the 1930s in Jamaica and Dominica. The faith was inspired by two men, Marcus Garvey who founded the Back to Africa movement and Ras Tafari who became Emperor Haile Selassie of Ethiopia in 1930. The Emperor is considered to be the Messiah who will lead all black people to freedom. White culture and Christianity are not adhered to. There is a personal approach to the religion and individuals generally make their own way in life. The Old and New Testaments have been retained by the faith and Rastafarians believe that they are the true Jews who will eventually return to Africa and their true home.

Churches for worship do not exist and there are no official clergy. All followers are committed to a deep love of God and consider the body to be a temple. Traditional medical treatments may be rejected in favour of herbal or alternative therapies. Clothes which are considered to be second-hand are taboo and this will include hospital cotton gowns, the offer of which may be refused. Hair is worn long and in a dreadlock style which is very distinctive and a symbol of pride. A puritan ethic sustains personal dignity.

Postmortem examination

The suggestion of a postmortem examination would be met with some distaste by Rastafarians. However, consistent with its mantra, the Rastafarian religion leaves the final decision up to the individual.

Funerals

There is no elaborate ritual involved in the funeral of a Rastafarian believer. Burial would be preferred over cremation, but again the choice is left to the individual.

Sikhism

A Sikh is a follower of Guru Nanak and his succeeding nine Gurus who are regarded as saints. In 1469 Guru Nanak combined Islam and Hinduism to take the best aspects of both religions. Sikhs believe in one God and follow the holy book of the Guru Grant Sahab which is a collection of the writings of the ten Gurus. To a Sikh, all people are equal and the responsibility for worship rests with the individual. *Amrit* is a form of confirmation which is adopted by some Sikhs, binding them to observe special rules.

RELIGIOUS ASPECTS
— Religions & Cultures

A male Sikh is given the honorary title of 'Singh', while the females are given the title 'Kaur'. Both were introduced in 1699 and mean 'lion' and 'princess' respectively.

Termination of pregnancy

There is no formal objection to the termination of a pregnancy.

Funerals

The body of a baby should be given to the parents to perform the normal funeral rites. The Sikh custom is to cremate the body of the deceased (a baby may be buried) and this would take place within 24 hours if possible. The coffin is usually taken to the family home and opened for a short time to allow the relatives and friends to view the body. After brief prayers the coffin is accompanied to the Sikh temple or *gurdwara* for more prayers. If cremation is considered and ashes are available from the crematorium, they are usually scattered on a river or in the sea. Sometimes ashes are taken to the River Sutle at Anandpur in the Punjab where Sikhism was founded.

Non-believers

It is necessary for health professionals to understand the difference in extremes of non-believers. A non-believer may be totally opposed to any suggestion of religious comfort but, again, the nurse, midwife or doctor has to approach each woman as an individual who may not behave as expected for their stated faith. The following are four examples of non-believers.

An atheist does not believe in the existence of a God or gods. This may then manifest in a total rejection of specific dogmas or a scepticism of all religious claims. An agnostic holds the view that humans can never be certain about issues relating to religious knowledge such as the existence of God. Since the sixteenth century the word 'humanism' has been applied to a person of entirely non-religious beliefs and values. Marxism is an example of a form of humanism. There are no set doctrines that humanists follow and their choice of 'cause' is held as the most important aspect of their beliefs and values. 'Causes' may vary from humanist to humanist. Belief in an 'open-mind' and an 'open-society' may be foremost concerns of a particular 'cause'.

As far as caring for a couple with no stated religious belief is concerned, it is still essential for the health professional to avoid making any assumptions. A long-lost faith may be rekindled during a traumatic event and it is important that the individual is allowed to explore their own response to the grief which they suffer.

CONCLUSION

The overwhelming message when confronted by an unfamiliar religious belief is to ask. Questions arising from interest and a willingness to do the right thing will always be welcome. For the couple, the opportunity to fulfil their individual rituals and customs may provide enormous support and strength for the months ahead. The ability to avoid making assumptions is also critical to the provision of good quality care. Treating each person as an individual with their own needs is the foundation for nursing and midwifery today. Religion is as crucial in this assessment as physical requirements. Help can be found in many sources, from official organisations to the ward orderly who happens to be of the same religious faith. The key is never to presume, always to ask.

REFERENCES

Dhammarati D (1989) Buddhist funerals. *Raft: The Journal of the Buddhist Hospital Trust* 1: 3.

Green J (1994) *Death with Dignity*. London, Nursing Times.

Hennells JR (1984) *Dictionary of Religions*. London, Penguin Reference Books.

Hospital Chaplaincies Council (1993) *Our Ministry and Other Faiths*, Sect. 1. London, Orphans Press.

Jacobs J (1994) *Guidance for Hospitals on the Care of Jewish Patients*. The Office of the Chief Rabbi, Adler House, Tavistock Square, London WC1H 9HN, UK.

Kohn I & Moffitt P-L (1994) Finding solace in your religion. In *Pregnancy Loss*, chap. 10, pp 138–153. London, Hodder Headline.

Lothian Racial Equality Council (1992) A guide to patients' beliefs and customs for health service staff. In *Religions and Cultures*. Edinburgh, Lothian Racial Equality Council.

Mander R (1994) Caring for the grieving mother. In *Loss and Bereavement in Childbearing*, chap. 4, pp 56–74. London, Blackwell Scientific.

Office of the Chief Rabbi (1994) *Stillbirth and Neonatal Death*. The Office of the Chief Rabbi, Adler House, Tavistock Square, London WC1H 9HN, UK.

Sampson C (1982) Some cultural aspects of care of patients. In *The Neglected Ethic*, chap. 3, pp 15–46. Maidenhead, McGraw-Hill.

Smith N (1993) Guidelines in pastoral care for clergy and hospital chaplains. In *Miscarriage, Stillbirth and Neonatal Death*. Joint Committee for Hospital Chaplaincy. London, Ludo Press.

RELIGIOUS ASPECTS
– Religions & Cultures

Stewart A & Dent A (1994) Multiracial issues. In (A Stewart & A Dent, eds) *At a Loss*, chap. 9, pp 184–192. London, Baillière Tindall.

Sucitto V (1989) Buddhist funerals. *Raft: The Journal of the Buddhist Hospital Trust* **1**: 1–3.

Chapter Eight

Funeral Arrangements

*That was one reason why the funeral was so important to us.
It marked his life not only to us but for our family, it created
memories, it forged bonds and it allowed people to express
their love to us.*

(Hall 1989)

A funeral offers those who are grieving an opportunity to say
goodbye. It can help to make the event a reality and allow people
to express their thoughts and feelings about the deceased (Worden
1992). Arrangements have to be made to dispose of the body either
through burial or cremation. In the case of a baby born dead or
who dies soon after birth the situation is the same: responsibility
has to be taken for ensuring that the remains are disposed of in a
dignified and respectful manner. The parent(s), for whom this may
be their first close encounter with death, may find the choices
confusing. The funeral can be arranged by the hospital or privately
by the family, except in the case of a neonatal death when the
responsibility rests with the family. Information about the options
available needs to be given to the mother and she then chooses
whom to discuss it further with. A contact telephone number given
on discharge will enable her to keep in touch during the decision-
making time. The funeral of the dead baby is an important aspect
of the grieving process; the decision has to be one which the
mother and father are both in agreement with and are sure that
they will not regret later.

Questions regarding funeral arrangements can be daunting
for the health professional. There are few resources within the
hospital to accommodate requests for further information. If the
hospital employs a Bereavement Administrator, the situation will
be much easier as that person will be responsible for guiding the
family through most of the practicalities. The midwife may wish to
attend the funeral and can check with the family whether this will
be acceptable.

The purpose of this chapter is to outline the choices which
are available to parents. Simply to say that one can choose

between cremation and burial is to abdicate one's duty to those parents. Gestational age, local agreements, hospital interpretations of policy documents, religious and cultural beliefs, documentation and so forth can all contribute to a confusing array of options and restrictions, from which the parents are expected to make an informed choice. The staff have a responsibility to try to ensure that parents are able to make that choice.

PRE-VIABLE BABIES

A pre-viable baby of less than 24 weeks gestation is not legally recognised unless there were signs of life at the time of delivery. Over the last decade attention has turned to the disposal arrangements for these babies. In the majority of hospitals, incineration or maceration were the only choices available. Concerns were voiced about the inappropriateness of these actions and there has been increasing recognition of the need to acknowledge perinatal loss and the importance of adequate mourning for all babies, regardless of gestational age. The publication of the Polkinghorne Report in 1989 brought attention to the research use of fetuses and fetal material.

The report summarised one aspect of its specific proposals thus:

> *On the basis of its potential to develop into a human being, a fetus is entitled to respect, according it a status broadly comparable to that of a living person.*

(Polkinghorne 1989)

In December 1991 the National Health Service Management Executive published a circular reiterating the statement and further adding:

> *That respect is due no matter what the circumstances of the loss (i.e. stillbirth, miscarriage or termination of pregnancy).*

(Department of Health 1991)

The Institute of Burial and Cremation Administration published a policy document in March 1992 as a response to the increasing demand for appropriate disposal arrangements for pre-viable fetuses (Institute of Burial and Cremation Administration 1992). On 1 October 1992 the legal age of viability was reduced from 28 to 24 weeks gestation. In consequence, statute law does not permit any form of registration for babies who do not exhibit signs of life at delivery. In 1992 the publication of *A Dignified Ending* drew attention to the importance of offering choice: primarily to the parents in respect of the disposal of the body or remains and, secondly, in requesting that the hospital policy deal with the issue of disposal in a dignified and respectful manner (Kohner 1992).

In order for this to be achieved, hospital policy has to recognise the significance of each baby born. The negotiation of contractual agreements is usually performed by staff outside the immediate department. They have to be fully informed of the requirements of the contract in order to ensure that it meets the client needs. It is important that liaison with the obstetricians and senior midwives takes place before the contract is signed. On the part of the funeral director there is very little benefit in signing a contract for the disposal of pre-viable fetuses as the funeral is usually performed free of charge or for a very minimal rate. The purchasing authority may include the appropriate disposal of all babies as a service specification when agreeing the contract with the provider unit.

For the parents of a pre-viable fetus born as a result of a spontaneous abortion, an intrauterine death or a therapeutic termination the choices are to allow the hospital to make the arrangements for incineration, burial or cremation or to choose to arrange the burial or cremation privately. There may be a request from the family to see and hold the baby and staff can encourage this if the remains are intact. As with all identifiable babies the taking of photographs is recommended, even if the family refuse to have them initially; by storing them in the casenotes staff can reassure the mother that, if she changes her mind they will be there for a number of years. Once the baby has been transferred to the mortuary, the same guidelines on viewing should apply as to all relatives of deceased patients.

Historically the disposal of the fetal remains was always the hospital's responsibility. The incineration or maceration of the fetus was conducted according to hospital guidelines and the parents were often unaware of the procedure, indeed the consensus view appeared to be that it was not necessary for the parents to be involved in the decision-making process. This attitude was not as coldhearted or as unfeeling as it appears; as with many aspects of the management of perinatal loss over the years, the disposal issue was approached with the intention to offer the least upset to the parents. Insight into the needs of the bereaved parents has revealed much about the importance of the funeral in the grieving process (Worden 1992).

Having recognised the inappropriateness of some methods of disposing of fetal remains, hospitals have moved away from incineration and maceration. Disposal arrangements tend to be with a local funeral director and the mother is aware of the method of disposal. But there can be occasions when the mother

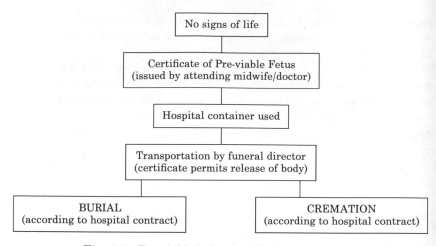

Fig. 8.1   Pre-viable baby: hospital arrangements.

leaves hospital without being involved in the decision about cremation or burial of her pre-viable baby. In this situation the mortuary cannot release the body to the funeral director and must hold the baby until permission has been sought from the parents. A clear training need for all members of staff is how the hospital disposes of fetal remains. The woman who attends the Accident & Emergency Department, has a spontaneous abortion, is admitted overnight for an evacuation of her uterus and is then discharged may slip through the net. The possibility of a breakdown in communication is increased when she is receiving care in more than one ward area. With sensitive issues which are not easy to discuss there may be a greater tendency to presume that someone else will have talked to her about it. Clear documentation in the casenotes will ensure that mistakes are rare. Written guidelines may be included in the ward procedure book or individual handbooks, and locum or agency staff have a responsibility to know local procedures when they are handling these situations. If the woman is discharged and has not been involved, it may be necessary for permission to be sought later; the GP may be approached or a midwife working in the area may contact her and visit.

Hospital Arrangements

Burial

A contractual agreement is required between the Health Authority, the Hospital trust and the local authority in order for the burial of pre-viable babies to take place. A collective space may be set aside such as the Babies Memorial Garden in Carlisle cemetery (West KJ 1994, personal communication). Once the space has been identified, arrangements are made with the hospital mortuary for a collection of babies at regular intervals. Except for multiple pregnancies, an individual, identified container is required for each baby. Local arrangements will vary and in some areas a shared grave will be used, while in others individual plots are allocated (Institute of Burial and Cremation Administration 1992). The idea of a shared grave may upset some parents and they may prefer to make alternative arrangements, but discovering this fact after the funeral is too late. Informing the parents of the date for the funeral and whether they can place flowers or can erect a remembrance stone is good practice.

Cremation

The cremation of tiny babies on an individual basis can be expensive for the crematorium. Local arrangements may be made to collect an agreed number at regular intervals. The furnace can then be fired up for a session and each coffin cremated separately according to the Institute of Burial and Cremation guidelines for good practice (Institute of Burial and Cremation Administration

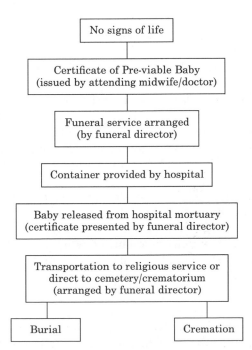

Fig. 8.2 Pre-viable baby: private arrangements.

1992). The cost of the crematorium for these sessions is covered by a contractual agreement with the hospital or with the local authority. The family should know the date and time of the cremation. Owing to the softness of fetal bones, special equipment is required to produce ashes; only a small amount of ashes will be left and the session will include the cremation of more than one baby. If the parents wish to have ashes, the crematorium will try to oblige but will inform the parents of the above.

Private Arrangements

At the outset of a pregnancy, arranging a funeral for a dead baby is the farthest thing from the minds of the prospective parents. If the horror becomes a reality, they will require clear, concise information about how to make the necessary arrangements. The parents may come up with their own suggestions which the staff are unaccustomed to – the request to take the baby home for a period before the burial, or to actually bury the baby in their garden.

Burial

Burying a baby in a private garden is perfectly feasible (see Burial on Private Land). The parents may approach the local funeral director to make the necessary arrangements and ensure that their wishes are attended to. By law there is no legal recognition of a pre-viable fetus and the funeral director can legitimately refuse to be involved. The hospital staff can warn the parents of this possibility and encourage them to try alternative funeral directors. Funerals can be conducted by a funeral director who is not local. The cost of a funeral for a baby is generally very low; in some areas no charge is made, for others there is the minimum local cemetery or crematorium charge to cover. If the parents have specific requests, the funeral director will advise on the additional costs imposed.

The parents may wish to arrange the funeral themselves. There is no difficulty with this; staff should advise them to contact the local cemetery or crematorium direct. Advice will be offered on the necessary forms which are required, when the funeral can take place and how to transport the baby. The hospital should be in a position to supply a suitable container.

Cremation

If a funeral director is involved, the arrangements with the local crematorium will be dealt with. The parents will need to decide on a suitable date and any additional requests which they may have.

The availability of ashes needs to be clear; the parents can then decide what they would like to do with them. If a funeral director is not involved, the parents will have to liaise with the crematorium personally. Advice will be required on how to transport the baby; a suitable container should be provided by the hospital.

Hospital and Private Arrangements

Container

A separately identified container must be used for each fetus, the only exception to this being multiple pregnancies (Department of Health 1991; Institute of Burial and Cremation Administration 1992; Kohner 1992). A selection of sizes should be available in the hospital mortuary or from the funeral director. The parent(s) can decide whether to dress the baby or to place personal items such as a teddy bear in the coffin.

Documentation

When a pre-viable baby is born, any nurse, doctor or midwife who was present can sign a Certificate of Pre-viable Fetus. Although the certificate is not a legal requirement, it is a response to the changing practice of disposal arrangements for these babies. In the days of incineration or maceration as the only choice available, the baby remained the property of the hospital. As soon as the arrangements indicate that the remains may be removed from the hospital premises to a chapel of rest, a cemetery, a crematorium or a private dwelling, a release form is required to obtain the baby from the mortuary. The grey area within the law does not satisfy this requirement, so the Institute of Burial and Cremation Adminstration advised on the Certificate of Medical Practitioner or Midwife (Institute of Burial and Cremation Administration 1992). The parents may be given this form to hand to the funeral director or to the mortuary and the baby will be released.

The crematorium will always require completed forms. It is advisable for the staff to ensure that the necessary form is completed by the required number of doctors at the time of delivery, particularly if the doctor was not a regular member of staff. If the mother decides to have the baby buried, the cremation form can simply be discarded.

Burial

- Certificate of Pre-viable Fetus (from ward staff)
- Routine application for burial form (from cemetery or funeral director)

Cremation
- Certificate of Pre-viable Fetus (from ward staff)
- Application for cremation
- Authority to cremate

The family may request a copy of the Certificate of Pre-viable Fetus as a memento of the baby and a recognition of his or her existence. The staff can assist in this matter by photocopying the original.

Transport

The baby will be stored in the hospital mortuary while the funeral arrangements are being made, and can then be moved to a chapel of rest within the funeral home. The family will be able to visit the baby if they so wish; it may be possible for them to stay overnight. Alternatively, they may choose to take the baby home until the funeral. This custom is less frequently performed today, possibly because death is not so acceptable or confronted so often as in the days when mortality rates were higher. The use of the front parlour for receiving the body of the deceased encouraged the recognition of the bereaved by neighbours and family who visited the home. Few houses or flats today have the additional space and the coffin may have to be placed in the centre of the living area or a bedroom. The room temperature has to be regulated to prevent rapid decomposition. The growth of the number of funeral parlours offers an alternative and visiting the body at the chapel of rest or funeral home may be preferable to all involved.

The funeral director will recommend that the baby is embalmed, a process which is usually included in any cost for the funeral. The embalmer may visit the house and advise the family. If the body has not been embalmed it will deteriorate more rapidly; in these situations only one night at home would be recommended. If the coffin is open, a veil should be placed over the baby's face to protect it from flies (Albin B 1992, personal communication).

If a funeral director has been involved in the arrangements he or she will take responsibility for all transporting of the body. As the coffin will be so small a separate hearse is rarely employed and the family travel in the same car. A platform can be used in the front of the car and the coffin is placed on this.

Mementos

As with all perinatal loss, remembering the baby will be very important to the mother and all other family involved. Regardless of how advanced the pregnancy was, she will not forget the loss. Photographs are a memento which provide lasting evidence that a baby existed, a fact which she may doubt in the years ahead. Involving siblings in the photographic session may require some sensitive encouragement by the staff and, ultimately, the decision will rest with the parent(s). The same rules as with photographs of term babies apply – attention to background detail and the position of the baby. Secure storage of unwanted photographs should ensure that they do not fall out of the casenotes in the years ahead.

A hospital-arranged funeral will not include religious content. A Service of Remembrance may be held within the hospital chapel and parents are invited to attend. In addition an annual service may be performed which is open to all bereaved parents over an undefined period of time. The aim of the service is to meet the needs of all bereaved families, regardless of their personal religious beliefs. A representative from each of the local churches may be involved in the service. The hospital staff are also invited to attend and it is an opportunity to be reunited with some of the parents they have cared for over the years.

Planting a tree or rosebush in memory of a dead baby can be done in a local park or cemetery. The grounds of the hospital may also be suitable. Permission can be sought from the local authority or the hospital administrator. A small plaque bearing details of the child may be placed at the site.

In some instances parents may wish to make a donation to the hospital and require information about how to do this. The recipient department will use the money to purchase a suitable item such as a Moses basket or a rocking chair. Recognition in the form of a thank-you letter and, if appropriate, an inscription on the equipment will thank the family in return.

STILLBIRTHS AND NEONATAL DEATHS

Confusion regarding neonatal deaths may arise if the pregnancy has not reached 24 weeks. Recognition of a live birth may be difficult for the staff to contemplate if the baby only lived for a minute or so following the birth. In situations which are arbitrary, the midwife or doctor is wise to seek the advice of a consultant paediatrician for clarification. It is important that the mother receives consistent information regarding her child. Staff who are concerned about the stress of 'inflicting' a distressing episode of registering the baby should remember that the registration process clearly identifies the baby as a person rather than a miscarriage.

The significance of this may be very important to the mother and her partner and assist in the grieving process.

Hospital Arrangements

Stillborn babies are not permitted to be incinerated and must be buried or cremated. A neonatal death is the responsibility of the family and the arrangements cannot be left to the hospital.

Burial

Local arrangements between hospital trusts, health authorities and cemeteries or crematoriums have been working since 1975. Although they are not involved in the direct arrangements for the burial, parents should be informed of the date and time, where the grave will be and whether the plot is shared with other babies. The

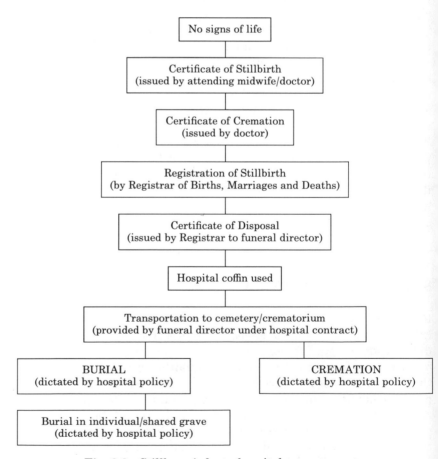

Fig. 8.3 Stillborn infants: hospital arrangements.

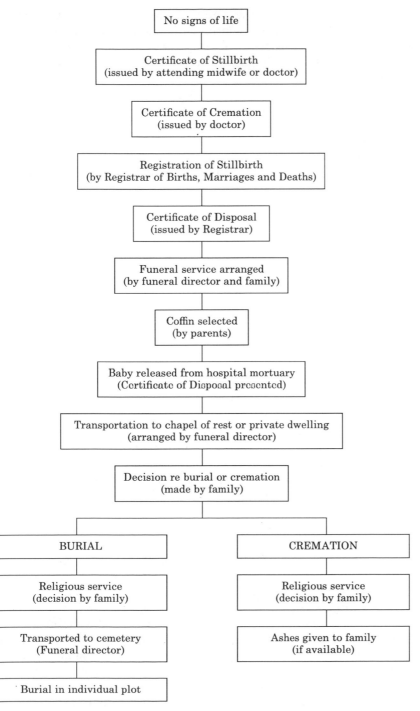

Fig. 8.4   Stillborn infants: private arrangements.

latter is likely to be the case, and this may change some parents' minds. The identified area mentioned in the section on pre-viable babies may also apply. Knowing that they can mark the grave in some way may be very important to the couple but it may not be a question they think to ask.

Cremation

The contractual arrangement held by the hospital may include cremation as an option. The same rules apply regarding informing the family about the timing and the availability of ashes as with a pre-viable baby.

Private Arrangements

Burial

Private arrangements for the burial can be confusing if the parents do not involve a funeral director. The death of a baby is often the first close encounter for a couple where they are the main organisers of the burial. Help from an experienced funeral director can be very reassuring and the couple can be encouraged to choose the most appropriate burial. In the absence of a funeral director, the mother or her partner will need to liaise directly with the crematorium or cemetery.

A plot for burial may offer three choices: an adult grave which may be used in the future for other family members, a private child-size plot in an identified area of the cemetery, or an existing family grave. The opportunity to choose should be clear to the mother. Knowing that her baby is beside other children may offer some comfort, or using a grave where other loved ones have been buried can be reassuring.

Choice in the type of funeral service which is held may be very important to the couple. The funeral director can work with the religious leader to ensure the wishes of the family are carried out. The difficulty of holding a religious service for a baby is in the lack of suitable material to use – all the more reason for tailoring the service to the individual family's needs and beliefs (Knowles 1994). The coffin may be open and the baby on view during the ceremony, or the baby may be held by a member of the family and only placed in the coffin at the end of the service. Expectations of a funeral can restrict personal choice, so the parents may be put off suggesting their ideas because of other people's views of what is suitable. A sympathetic cleric or funeral director can help to overcome this.

Cremation

Again a funeral director may not be involved in the proceedings, although the same advice regarding help applies. The parents need to have information about the time and date.

Hospital and Private Arrangements

Container

Choosing a coffin which is appropriate to the person who has died can be hard; for a baby the choice may be very limited. If the hospital has responsibility for the arrangements, a single type of coffin will be available in a variety of sizes (this may restrict what the parents can place in the casket). For private use the coffin will be made of composition board covered with white fabric, wood veneer, oak, mahogany, elm or beech. The inside will be lined with a suitable material (Albin 1992, personal communication). In the case of a multiple pregnancy the babies may be placed in the same container.

Transport

The transporting arrangements will be the same as with a pre-viable baby. The baby may be taken home and embalming is increasingly being advised.

Burial on private land

The request to take the dead baby home and bury him or her in the garden is an unusual one. It is not an option which many parents consider, yet if the request is made the staff need to be able to provide information on how to arrange a 'green' burial. Any adult, child or baby (including stillbirths and pre-viable babies) may be buried or have their ashes scattered on private land. Although practices have moved away from incineration or maceration of dead babies, the general public are not always aware of changes. Reliance on relatives and friends for information may mean the woman receives outdated ideas from those persons' personal experience in the past. The midwife or nurse is wise to check that the woman is making an informed choice and knows all the options available. The author has been in the situation of receiving a midnight telephone call from the gynaecology ward requesting guidance over a woman who wished to bury her 16-week baby in the garden. Reassured that she did not want to do so at that precise moment, we discussed her choices the following morning before she was discharged. She had been under the impression that all babies were 'sluiced', as she termed it, and

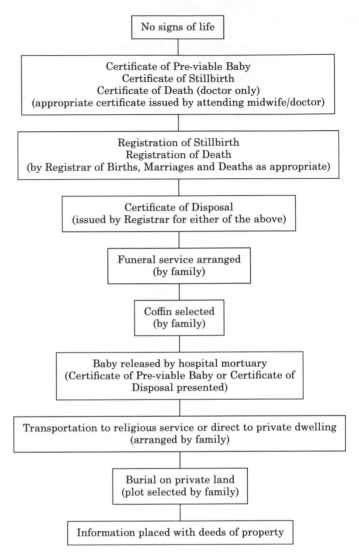

Fig. 8.5 All babies: burial on private land.

wanted something more dignified for her baby. She had reached this conclusion by remembering the media coverage from years ago of aborted fetuses left in sluices. We provided here with information about the reality of disposal arrangements and reassured her that her baby would be safe in the hospital mortuary while she made her choice. Two days later she asked for the hospital to arrange the burial.

If the parents choose burial in the garden because they consider it to be most suitable for their baby, certain factors must be taken into account:

- The baby or fetal remains must be placed in a suitable, identified container. Containers can be obtained from the hospital or a funeral director.
- For neonatal deaths and stillbirths the registration process must have been completed.
- The baby may be transported by private car. In case of accidents the local police may require details of the journey.
- If the baby is taken to a private dwelling before the funeral, consideration must be given to the storage conditions.
- The burial should be at a suitable distance from water supplies (50 metres is recommended for adults) (Albery et al 1993). The depth should be 2 metres (6 feet). A suitable site would have no water at the bottom of the grave when dug.
- Information about the grave should be stored with the house deeds. Legally there are no requirements to inform the Environmental Health Officer or the local authority. Planning permission is not required.
- The presence of the grave may devalue the house by as much as 30%; advice should be sought from the local authority on this issue.
- Neighbours, especially if they overlook the garden, may object to the grave.
- A plaque or tombstone may be erected in the garden.
- A direct licence from a Secretary of State is required to exhume the body. This does not apply to pre-viable babies who are not legally recognised.
- Burial in nature reserves is possible in a few places such as Harrogate and Carlisle. Private nature reserve burial grounds are also being planned.
- There is no limit to the number of burials which can take place on private land. English law does not define a cemetery as having a particular number of graves within it.

Cost

The cost of a funeral for a baby will depend on the local arrangement. Many funeral directors will not charge anything for a basic funeral; charges are made for extra cars or requests which are outside the basic service. Families on social security may be entitled to the Social Fund; this provides help with the cost of the funeral and additional costs, e.g. for particular religious observations (DHSS 1989). Funerals can be expensive and an

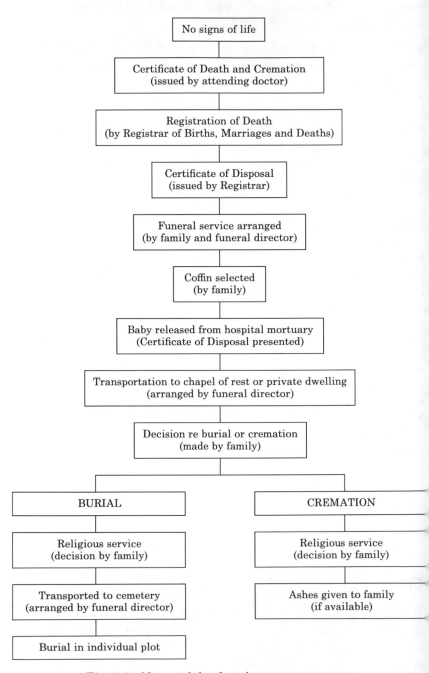

Fig. 8.6   Neonatal death: private arrangements.

experienced funeral director will advise the family to consider the request they are making. In the immediate grieving period there may be a temptation to spend beyond one's means; wise counsel is helpful.

Overseas Arrangements

If the stillbirth or death occurs outside the United Kingdom, arrangements can be made to fly the body home. Equally, a baby born here may be transported overseas; a funeral director will make the arrangements. Costs will vary according to need.

CONCLUSION

The funeral often marks the beginning of the mourning period. The bereaved may focus on the practical issues surrounding the death, but when the service is over the finality of the loss becomes a reality. To the parents of a dead baby, arranging the funeral may be the only opportunity to 'do something' for their child. It may also provide one of the few mementoes which they have to keep. The role of the health professional is to assist the family to make the right choice for them, one which they will be happy with for the future. Uncertainty and confusion are not unusual in these circumstances, and staff must do all they can to ensure that the family receive the correct advice and are put in touch with the right people.

FUNERAL ARRANGEMENTS
– Stillbirths & Neonatal
Deaths

REFERENCES

Albery N, Elliot G & Elliot J (1993) *Natural Death Handbook: A Manual for Improving the Quality of Living and Dying*. London, Natural Death Centre.

Department of Health (1991) *Sensitive Disposal of the Dead Fetus and Fetal Tissue* EL (91) 144, 12 December 1991.

DHSS (1989) Help when someone dies. In *A Guide to Social Security Benefits*. London, HMSO.

Hall J (1989) Mourning for Philip. *Good Housekeeping* Apr.: 129–131.

Institute of Burial and Cremation Administration (1992) *The Disposal of Fetal Remains: A Policy Document*. March.

Knowles S (1994) A passage through grief: The Western Australian Rural Pregnancy Loss Team. *British Medical Journal* **309**: 1705–1708.

Kohner N (1992) Recommendations for good practice in the disposal of the bodies and remains of babies born dead before the legal age of viability. *A Dignified Ending*. London, SANDS.

Polkinghorne J (1989) Conclusions: Summary of principles. In *Review of the Guidelines on the Research Use of Fetuses and Fetal Remains*, p. 20. London, HMSO.

Worden JW (1992) *Grief Counselling and Grief Therapy*, pp 61–62. London, Tavistock Publications.

Chapter Nine

Support

Support following the death of a baby before delivery is needed, not only for the grieving mother and family but for everyone involved. News of a perinatal death has a tendency to spread rapidly through the department; it affects other clients, ancillary and domestic staff as well as the professionals. The *Oxford English Dictionary* defines support as 'to give strength to, to enable to last or to continue'. Every single day in the hospital environment will produce scenes where doctors, nurses and midwives are called upon to support their clients. They may become very skilled at providing support but are not so efficient when it comes to meeting their own needs. Who cares for the carers? The purpose of this chapter is to consider the needs of the staff, to look at the ways support can be provided and how to encourage doctors, nurses and midwives to accept the concept of help in caring for each other.

TRAINING

Tschudin comments that 'charity begins at home, so does support. Before anyone can support another person, he or she needs to be supported' (Tschudin 1991). Time is not built into busy work schedules to allow a breathing space for staff, there is always another client to be seen, a clinic which is running late, another client to admit on delivery suite, more paperwork to complete, and so on.

From their first introduction to the subject of obstetrics and midwifery, students need to understand that death occurs within this speciality. They must be encouraged to appreciate that death is not a spectre to be scared of, that handled sensitively it can be a positive experience for all concerned. Attention may be turned to consider their own response to death – how do they cope with it? Is the death of a patient a failure on their part? Students need to recognise that, for some patients, death can be a welcome relief. In obstetrics this may be evident if the parents have decided to continue a pregnancy where there is a known fetal abnormality.

The baby may eventually die, but offering choice to the parents enables them to live with their conscience and know that they made the right decision for them.

Tutorials and lectures need to address how to deal with the loss of a baby in various circumstances. The support which is available to the parents should be discussed; groups such as the Stillbirth and Neonatal Death Society (SANDS) are generally willing to speak to groups of students and explain their role. The response of a bereaved couple can be one of aggression and this may be directed at the staff involved in their care, a disturbing experience for students to witness. Communication is vital to allow the students to cope with their own fears and reactions; time to sit down and talk with the staff or a personal tutor should be encouraged.

An inability to acknowledge death in a personal sense within a society which rejects death generally may result in doctors who compensate for interaction by using distancing tactics (Black et al 1989) to detach themselves from the reality of the person behind the grief and to hide behind the technical elements of the role. Medical, nursing and midwifery education teaches the tools for the trade; invariably attention is paid to the 'bedside manner', but mainly the focus is on the technical attributes. Until they enter the clinical area and meet a 'patient' the human element of the role may escape the would-be doctor. For midwifery and nursing students the reality of caring for real people comes earlier. Carers need to be emotionally secure themselves in order to provide optimal care and support (Mander 1994). In contradiction to the concept of the doctor, nurse or midwife's professional purpose, death may be seen as a failure and may generate guilt (Black et al 1989; Mander 1994). Doctors may have particular trouble with this aspect as they are haunted by the image of the healer – to be a doctor is to cure. Failure to cure may mean failure as a doctor and therefore acceptance of the ultimate 'failure', death, can be very difficult.

In the United States medical schools recognised the need to include courses on death and dying in the 1960s; by 1980 only 10 colleges were not including something on the curriculum. Medical schools in this country have caught up and by 1983 only 4 out of 62 were not running a programme (Black et al 1989). The content of these sessions can vary enormously.

Role play can be used to help students observe and understand their own behaviour. Careful preparation and facilitation is required to ensure that the session is controlled and the 'debrief' takes place. A number of scenarios may be used; for example, a scene may involve one student playing the doctor's role while another is the patient who is informed that he has six months to live. The other students observe the action and comment on the interaction between the two. The participants are given the opportunity to describe their own feelings and to step out of the role at the end. With the use of video equipment the role play can be replayed and commented upon (Black et al 1989). An alternative to using the students for both parts would be to hire actors for one of the roles. The actress may be the midwife while the student midwife is the expectant mother; the scenario reveals that the client has just been diagnosed with an intrauterine death. Feedback from these sessions is vital but must be handled appropriately. The unknown personal experience of the student may be a very sensitive and unexplored area. Exposing an unrecognised emotion may cause problems unless it is dealt with appropriately (Mander 1994).

POST-BASIC EDUCATION

Midwifery as a profession has always recognised the importance of ongoing education. A mandatory course of instruction is required on a five-year basis and a notification of intention to practise by each midwife records this information (UKCC 1993a). We, as professionals, are good at what we are trained to do; we practise what we have been taught and we improve. If we have not had the exposure to a situation or had the opportunity to become good, we may seek to avoid revealing our inexperience or deficiency (Mander 1994).

Ongoing debate exists about the need for preceptors for qualified staff. The current views are that newly qualified midwives are in need of a period of support for four months, while the opposing argument is that midwives are trained to take on the responsibility of their own action at the point of registration (Jackson 1994, 1995). With the introduction of Post-registration Education and Practice (PREP) in 1993, the United Kingdom Central Council for Nursing, Midwifery and Health Visiting (UKCC) considered the provision of support and preceptorship to be necessary for all midwives, nurses and health visitors (UKCC 1993b).

While the discussion continues, some areas of support are easily identifiable. The support offered by more senior and/or more experienced midwives towards colleagues caring for their first stillbirth is often unsung. Strength is gained from the knowledge that the other midwives are aware that this case is different, with challenges of a very individual nature and a need to share feelings and fears.

Preceptorship may be implemented as a formal process; alternatively, the newly qualified midwife chooses his or her own. The important factor is that the support is there and that she or he does not carry their own grief of the situation around with them. The death of a baby is different from that of an adult or even a child; the process of birth is associated with life, and recognition of the fact that perinatal mortality occurs does not make it easier to accept that the process has failed (Worden 1992).

Reactions to caring for grieving and bereaved families may affect staff in different ways. For some, regular exposure to death may make them become immune to the worst kinds of suffering – in varying degrees enabling them to continue performing their roles. For others, the contact may have a personal cost and become a concern unless feelings can be dealt with.

The response of colleagues at this time is crucial. The avoidance of any blame for becoming 'too attached' or 'getting involved when he or she should know better' is important to the individual's survival of the emotional impact. There will always be the situation or client who affects the professional more deeply. The impact of this may be related to the circumstances of the loss, but it may also be about the doctor or nurse identifying with that person. The carer has losses and situations in his or her own personal life to deal with.

IMMEDIATE HELP

In the immediate environment of the ward area, a variety of 'amateur' help may be encountered, such as the coffee room counselling session with other members of staff on duty, sharing the stress and concerns about providing adequate care. A good manager will appreciate that staff work better if they are well supported in the work environment. There are many people within the structure who can provide support: the chaplain, managers, Supervisors of Midwives, senior doctors, peers, tutors, friends. Many hospitals now employ a full-time counsellor to help meet staff needs; the Occupational Health Department is always willing to listen.

Sometimes just the opportunity to sit down and reflect on a case is all that is required. For nurses and midwives this can be achieved over coffee break; doctors may find that the demands on their time, racing between clinics and operating theatres, preclude this breathing space. To stop and ask for help may be considered a weakness; no one wants to be seen as a failure in the eyes of their peers. It is important that any opportunity to discuss the case is used constructively and supportively.

Multidisciplinary sharing of support is important, recognition between the professions that we work together towards a common aim. Schott refers to the potential to be gained from the midwife's role in educating doctors, highlighting that the medical students of today are the obstetricians and GPs of the future. If we expect them to understand the process of 'normal' childbirth, then we must allow them in, encourage their involvement in our deliveries and teach them what the role of a midwife is. The wider scope which this covers is the ability to teach doctors about death. Invariably when a doctor encounters the death of a patient on a general ward, he or she leaves the bedside and the procedures to the nursing staff (Schott 1995). Sparing time to talk to relatives, the doctor is unlikely to appreciate the importance of sharing silence and a cup of tea with the bereaved. Nurses are accustomed to mopping up the tears, packing the belongings and ensuring that the grief-stricken relatives have transport home.

When a woman is in labour and her baby is already dead, she requires a lot of support and comfort from the staff around her. The doctor may need to be closely involved in her care, encountering her during long hours of labour. How does he or she know what to say or how to offer comfort? Usually by taking cues from the midwife in the room who may be unaware that she is a silent teacher.

SECONDARY SUPPORT

'Could I have done better?' is a question many health professionals ask themselves. The answer will vary according to the individual circumstances of the case: occasionally 'yes' and sometimes 'unknown'. Identifying the need to reflect and review the quality of care in hospitals is becoming increasingly popular. The role of clinical audit is increasing for all professions, including those allied to medicine.

To reflect on one's practice is a matter of learning from experience; there is much to be gained from sharing this with colleagues. Obviously there is a need to ensure that the process is handled properly. The manner in which information is shared about a particular case may vary from place to place. Depending on available time and facilities, the structure may be formal with regular meetings. Just as effective may be an ad hoc approach with discussion following a single event. The aim is to learn and build constructively with the benefit of hindsight. The main question is 'Could we have done anything differently?' Again, a multidisciplinary meeting may be the opportunity for shared

learning. The difficulty is in avoiding a 'witch hunt' with
individuals feeling that their practice is going to be criticised in
public. Staff may also be encouraged to keep reflective diaries
chronicling their working experience.

At the end of the shift or visit, the midwife, nurse or doctor
may be left emotionally drained from providing such stressful care.
Women recall with great clarity the events while they were in
hospital. The stress for the midwife is being depended upon to
support and provide comfort at a time when he or she has no
reserves of energy left (Greaves 1994). The worst time may be the
point of delivering the baby at the end of a long labour. Any
insensitivity will be noted and remembered by the woman; she
does not have the mental space to consider the stress placed on the
midwife. Communication is critical – for the midwife to admit to
being too tired and needing a break. Emphasis is placed on
continuity, but this must be a realistic standard.

The relationship between carer and client may continue for
some weeks. The draining effect this can have on the individual
midwife has to be recognised; midwives have stated the importance
of support from their manager at this time (Stewart and Dent
1994). As recognition grows of the need for support, so the network
grows. The introduction of a support group within a trust may
develop gradually, depending on recognised need. The initiative
will require support for its success, with commitment of time and
resources.

A successful support group needs clearly identified aims
and objectives in order to measure its progress. An individual is
unlikely to achieve a great deal with a group idea; a steering
group provides more impetus to get the idea off the ground and to
monitor it. As the majority of such groups will be internally
organised, the facilitator(s) will require some training in their role
(Kellet 1992). The group may meet over a series of weeks and
undertake a mini bereavement course. Emphasis could be placed
on the grief process, the effects on the parents and encouraging
the midwives to consider their own feelings (Sherratt 1987). A lack
of hierarchy is important within this group, as much can be learnt
from colleagues at all levels.

Inviting representatives from organisations such as
SANDS presents an opportunity for staff to appreciate the role
which these groups play in the months and years following the
loss. In addition to describing their organisation, the
representative may have a personal experience to relate; that
experience may have been some time ago and staff can learn a lot
from listening to the account. From it they can appreciate how far
health professionals working with SANDS, SATFA, etc. have
moved in helping the recently bereaved, but also understand how

much farther there is to go in this whole area (Roch 1987). If a representative from the organisation is not available, recommended reading for staff could include books which give account of parents' experiences, for example, *When a Baby Dies* (Kohner and Henley 1991).

LONG-TERM SUPPORT

The end of involvement with this particular client may be the end of the shift, or some weeks hence in the community setting. In between times the doctor, nurse or midwife will have carried on with their regular duties. Colleagues will forget the individual case as others take over. We recognise this fact by constantly stressing the importance of contemporaneous documentation on all clients. The assumption is that you will forget tomorrow the details of today's case, regardless of how well you know the woman. In certain circumstances the details are too deeply implanted on the professional's mind to ever be forgotten. The issue here is about support and how to move on. Delivering a dead baby is a very stressful experience. Every midwife is affected by the event; most use the experience positively but are not overwhelmed by it, a few find it hard to forget and are affected in their day-to-day practice. Recognition of ongoing grief in the professional is important; there may be other factors in their life which is contributing to this. Help and support from the various hospital staff already mentioned can prevent a long-term problem developing.

Before we get to the point of needing assistance to cope with unresolved grief in ourselves, we should be recognising the potential for it to occur. Looking after ourselves is a task we often fail to perform, given irregular working patterns, lack of sleep, juggling work with home and, possibly, children: all the inherent difficulties of fulfilling a very taxing job and coping with the outside world. How we, the health professionals, deal with stress is never very high on the agenda. Yet we are expecting a great deal from ourselves and our colleagues. The changing pattern of providing continuity and choice for clients presents its own set of unique problems. Are we fully equipped to support this family unit through this experience? Who can we share the load with? Continuity of carer is appreciated by the client, but the midwife may be totally exhausted by it. Committing oneself to being present for the birth rather than the duration of the shift requires a lot of energy. The midwife has to take care not to raise expectations too high and to be realistic in her approach to all her clients.

'Healer heal thyself' is not a rule which doctors, nurses and midwives abide by. Stewart suggests a combination of regular exercise, well-balanced meals, a relaxing hobby, knowing your stress signals and smiling at people. Above all, remember that the carers have choices too (Stewart and Dent 1994).

CONCLUSION

Undoubtedly there is much more which can be done to support the carer. Part of the problem is identifying those in need of support: the medical profession has not always appeared sympathetic to the idea of support for doctors. Nursing and midwifery has moved towards the idea of providing a staff counsellor in the last ten years. Gradually the attitude is changing and an acceptance of the incredible demands which caring for the sick and dying places on doctors and the associated professions is showing. Provision to meet these needs is still a long way from perfect. The thought that they are unable to cope in a crisis may still be foremost in many health professionals' minds when they find themselves in tears at the end of a shift. The reality is that they are responding in a way most lay people would recognise as expected when confronted by a terminally ill patient and distressed relatives. Sometimes just a few moments are required to regain the coping mechanism, time spent talking to colleagues or having a coffee break in peace.

REFERENCES

Black D, Hardoff D & Nelki J (1989) Educating medical students about death and dying. *Archives of Disease in Childhood* **64**: 750–753.

Greaves J (1994) Normal and abnormal grief reactions: Midwifery care after stillbirth. *British Journal of Midwifery* **2**: 61–65.

Jackson K (1994) Preceptorship involves irreconcilable concepts. *British Journal of Midwifery* **2**: 339.

Jackson K (1995) Do midwives need preceptors? *British Journal of Midwifery* **3**: 372–386.

Kellet J (1992) Facilitating support groups: A pilot study. *Nursing Standard* **6**: 23.

Kohner N & Henley A (1991) *When a Baby Dies*. London, Pandora Press.

Mander R (1994) Staff reactions and support. In *Loss and Bereavement in Childbearing*, pp 137–153. London, Blackwell Scientific Publications.

Roch S (1987) Sharing the grief. *Nursing Times* **83**: 52.

Schott J (1995) The midwife's role in educating doctors. *British Journal of Midwifery* **3**: 5–6.

Sherratt DR (1987) What do you say? *Midwives Chronicle and Nursing Notes*, **August**: 235–236.

Stewart A & Dent A (1994) Relevant issues of health workers. In
    (A Stewart & A Dent, eds) *At A Loss*, pp 193–205. London, Baillière
    Tindall.
Tschudin V (1991) *Counselling Skills for Nurses*, pp 13–20. London,
    Baillière Tindall.
UKCC (1993a) *Midwives' Rules*, Refresher Courses (Rule 37), p. 17. United
    Kingdom Central Council for Nursing, Midwifery and Health Visiting.
UKCC (1993b) *Registrar's Letter*, 4 January 1993. United Kingdom Central
    Council for Nursing, Midwifery and Health Visiting.
Worden JW (1992) *Grief Counselling and Grief Therapy*. London, Tavistock
    Publications.

SUPPORT
– Long-term Support

Appendix One

Resources

ORGANISATIONS

British Institute of Funeral Directors   146A High Street, Tonbridge, Kent TN9 1BB

Brook Advisory Centres   Central Office, 153A East Street, London SE1 2SD. Tel. 0171 7081234
Helps families and health workers after abortion. Centres located in cities; advice and contraceptive supplies to young people aged less then 25 years.

The Child Bereavement Trust   1 Hillside, Riversdale, Bourne End, Buckinghamshire SL8 5EB.
Offers video and book resources for bereaved families and training for professionals.

CHOICE   PO Box 20, Oxford. Tel. 01865 242333
Telephone counselling for women making a decision to have an abortion and afterwards.

Commission for Racial Equality   Elliot House, Allington Street, London SW1E 5EH. Tel. 0171 8287022

Compassionate Friends   53 North Street, Bristol BS3. Tel. 0117 953 9639
Support for parents, groups, leaflets.

CRUSE   126 Sheen Road, Richmond, Surrey TW9 1UR. Tel. 0181 9404818
Provides support to the bereaved by trained counsellors.

Foundation for the Study of Infant Deaths   35 Belgrave Square, London SW1X 8PS. Tel 0171 2350965
Provides befriending, local groups, information and leaflets and support research.

LIFE   Head Office, 7 Parade, Leamington Spa, Warwickshire CV32 4DG. Tel. 01926 311667
Organisation opposed to abortion; provides counselling and temporary accommodation for pregnant women.

London Bereavement Project Group   68 Chilton Street, London NW1 1JR. Tel 0171 3880241
Offers counselling on bereavement and Jewish counselling.

Loreene Hunte Foundation for Black Bereaved Families   11 Kingston Square, London SE19 1JE. Tel. 0171 7617728

Miscarriage Association   PO Box 2, Ossett, West Yorkshire WF5 9XG. Tel. 01945 830515
Provides local groups, befriending and information resources.

National Association of Funeral Directors   618 Warwick Road, Solihull, West Midlands B9 1AA

National Association for Maternal and Child Welfare   1 South Audley Street, London W1Y 6JS

National Council for Hospice and Specialist Palliative Care Services   59 Bryanston Street, London W1A 2AZ. Tel. 0171 6111153
Have appointed a worker responsible for identifying the issues related to black and ethnic minority communities.

Pregnancy Advisory Service   Central London Bureau, 11–13 Charlotte Street, London W1P 1HD. Tel. 0171 6378962
Centres throughout the country; provide pre- and post-abortion counselling, access to termination at less than 22 weeks.

The Stillbirth and Neonatal Death Society (SANDS)   28 Portland Place, London W1N 9XG. Tel. 0171 4365881
Support for parents whose babies are born dead or die soon after birth. Provides local groups, befriending and information resources. Also: 29–31 Euston Road, London NW1 2SD, Tel. 0171 8332851. They have appointed a worker who is responsible for looking at the needs of ethnic minority people.

Support After Termination for Fetal Abnormality (SAFTA)   29–30 Soho Square, London NW1V 6JB. Tel. 0171 2873752
Support group offering local contacts and some branches with befriending for couples. Organise a newsletter and have information resources. Produce a handbook for all parents making the decision to have a termination.

The Twins and Multiple Births Association (TAMBA) Bereavement Support Group   PO Box 30, Little Sutton, South Wirral L66 1TH. Tel. 0151 3480020
May have local contact, remembrance service, newsletter.

Women's Health and Reproductive Rights Information Centre   52–54 Feather Street, London EC1. Tel. 0171 2516332

Provide a whole range of information on different aspects of women's experience, including abortion and miscarriage. Can put women in contact with support groups.

LEAFLETS

Guide to postmortem examination – brief notes for parents and families who have lost a baby in pregnancy or early infancy, by the Department of Health, produced in consultation with the National Advisory Body for the Confidential Enquiry into Stillbirths and Deaths in Infancy, SANDS and FSID. Use the leaflet with parents as an aid to discussion.

VIDEOS AND TRAINING PACKAGES

An ache in their heart. For professionals and parents to equip them as companions for bereaved families. Resources include training sessions, handouts for families, children's books, a video, materials to form a memorial and medical information in layperson's language. Cost A$250. Yvonne Connelly, The University of Queensland, Department of Child Health, Clarence Court, Mater Children's Hospital, South Brisbane, Australia. Tel. 07 840 8154.

An introduction to Buddhism and *An introduction to Hinduism*, containing two audio cassettes, study guide and reading material. Open University, 1984. Available from the Learning Material Service, PO Box 188, Milton Keynes MK3 6HW.

Death at birth: two part video. This aims to help professionals understand parents' needs after loss of a baby, deal with their feelings and identify areas to improve practice. Produced by Jenni Thomas, Director of the Child Bereavement Trust.

Grief. Talks about different cultural reactions to grief and includes a sequence on a Vietnamese soldier being returned to his village for cremation. Good for starting a discussion. Distributed by Concord Films, 201 Felixstowe Road, Ipswich, Suffolk IP3 9BJ. Tel. 01473 726012.

The right to be understood, by Jane Shackman. A video and training pack on the employment and training of community interpreters. Available from the National Extension College, 18 Brooklands Avenue, Cambridge CB2 2HN. Tel. 01223 316644.

When our baby died: video and accompanying book, *Grieving after the death of your baby.* For parents and families and those who care for them. Produced by Jenni Thomas and Bradbury Williams. Written by Nancy Kohner. Professional Care Productions Ltd, 1 Millside, Riversdale, Bourne End, Bucks SL8 5EB.

Appendix Two

Documentation

ENGLAND AND WALES   Document

NORTHERN IRELAND

SCOTLAND

1A

MEDICAL CERTIFICATE OF STILL-BIRTH

(Births and Deaths Registration Act 1953, S.11(1), as amended by the Population (Statistics) Act 1960)
(Form prescribed by the Registration of Births and Deaths Regulations 1987)

SB 000000

To be given only in respect of a child which has issued forth from its mother after the 24th week of pregnancy and which did not at any time after being completely expelled from its mother breathe or show any other signs of life.

Registered at Entry No.

*I was present at the still-birth of a $\frac{\text{*male}}{\text{*female}}$ child born

*I have examined the body of a $\frac{\text{*male}}{\text{*female}}$ child which I am informed and believe was born

on _____ day of _____ 19___ to _____

(NAME OF MOTHER)

at _____

(PLACE OF BIRTH)

†{ 1 The certified cause of death has been confirmed by post-mortem.
2 Post-mortem information may be available later.
3 Post-mortem not being held.

Weight of fetus _____ grams
Estimated duration of pregnancy
State (a) the number of weeks of delivery
(b) When the child died
(i) before labour*
(ii) during labour*
(iii) not known*

*Strike out the words which do not apply.
†Ring appropriate digit.

CAUSE OF DEATH

a. Main diseases or conditions in fetus	
b. Other diseases or conditions in fetus	
c. Main maternal diseases or conditions affecting fetus	
d. Other maternal diseases or conditions affecting fetus	
e. Other relevant causes	

I hereby certify that (i) the child was not born alive, and
(ii) to the best of my knowledge and belief the cause of death and the estimated duration of pregnancy of the mother were as stated above.

Signature _____ Date _____

Qualification as registered by General Medical Council, or }
Registered No. as Registered Midwife. }

Address _____

For still-births in hospital: please give the name of the consultant responsible for the care of the mother

THIS IS NOT AN AUTHORITY FOR BURIAL OR CREMATION [SEE OVER]

1B

NOTE TO INFORMANT

Under Section 11(1) of the Births and Deaths Registration Act 1953, this certificate must be delivered to the Registrar of Births and Deaths by the person attending to give information of the particulars required to be registered concerning the still-birth. The persons qualified and liable to give such information include:

(1) the mother;

(2) the father (of a legitimate child only);

(3) the occupier of the house in which to the knowledge of that occupier the still-birth occurred;

(4) any person present at the still-birth;

(5) any person in charge of the still-born child;

(6) in the case of a still-born child found exposed, the person who found the child.

The still-birth is required to be registered within 42 days of its occurrence.

*Occupier in relation to a public institution includes the governor, keeper, master, matron, superintendent, or other chief resident officer.

2

MED B 0 9 5 5 5 9
1

Register to enter No. of Death Entry

BIRTHS AND DEATHS REGISTRATION ACT 1953

(Form prescribed by the Registration of Births, Deaths and Marriage (Amendment) (No. 2) Regulations 1985)

MEDICAL CERTIFICATE OF CAUSE OF DEATH OF A LIVE-BORN CHILD DYING WITHIN THE FIRST TWENTY-EIGHT DAYS OF LIFE

For use only by a Registered Medical Practitioner WHO HAS BEEN IN ATTENDANCE during the deceased's last illness, and to be delivered by him forthwith to the Registrar of Births and Deaths.

Name of child ....

Date of death .... day of .... 19 ...... Sex ....

Age at death .... days (complete period of 24 hours) .... hours

Place of death ....

Place of birth ....

Last seen alive by me .... day of .... 19 ......

1 The certified cause of death has been confirmed by post-mortem.

2 Information from post-mortem may be available later.

3 Post-mortem not being held.

4 I have reported this death to the Coroner for further action.

[See overleaf]

Please ring appropriate digit and letter.

a   Seen after death by me.

b   Seen after death by another medical practitioner but not by me.

c   Not seen after death by a medical practitioner.

CAUSE OF DEATH

SPECIMEN

a. Main diseases or conditions in infant ....

b. Other diseases or conditions in infant ....

c. Main maternal diseases or conditions affecting infant ....

d. Other maternal diseases or conditions affecting infant ....

e. Other relevant causes ....

I hereby certify that I was in medical attendance during the above named deceased's last illness, and that the particulars and cause of death above written are true to the best of my knowledge and belief.

Signature ....

Address ....

Qualifications as registered by General Medical Council ....

Date ....

For deaths in hospital   Please give the name of the consultant responsible for the above-named as a patient ....

3

ED 000000

CERTIFICATE OF REGISTRATION
OF BIRTH OR STILL-BIRTH

BIRTHS AND DEATHS REGISTRATION ACT 1953, s 12

(Form prescribed by the Registration of Births and Deaths Regulations 1987)

I, the undersigned, do hereby certify that the birth of

a $\frac{male^*}{female}$ *child (still-) born on the* ....

has been duly registered by me at Entry No .... *in Register No* ....

Name of informant ....

Qualification of informant ....

Date .... *Signature of registrar* ....

District .... *Sub-district* ....

*Strike out whichever does not apply.

Caution:—It is an offence to falsify a certificate or to make or knowingly use a false cer
or a copy of a false certificate intending it to be accepted as genuine to the prejudice of any p
or to possess a certificate knowing it to be false without lawful authority.

4

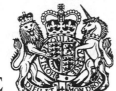

1 & 2 ELIZ. 2 CH. 20

GS143803

CERTIFICATE OF BIRTH

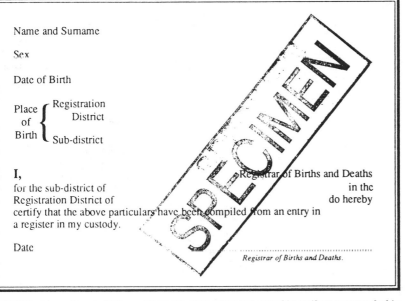

Name and Surname

Sex

Date of Birth

Place of Birth { Registration District

Sub-district

I,

for the sub-district of
Registration District of
certify that the above particulars have been compiled from an entry in
a register in my custody.

Registrar of Births and Deaths
in the
do hereby

Date

....
Registrar of Births and Deaths.

CAUTION – It is an offence to falsify a certificate or to make or knowingly use a false certificate or a copy of a false certificate intending it to be accepted as genuine to the prejudice of any person, or to possess a certificate knowing it to be false without lawful authority.

WARNING: THIS CERTIFICATE IS NOT EVIDENCE OF THE IDENTITY OF THE PERSON PRESENTING IT.

5

D. Cert.
R.B.D.

CERTIFIED COPY
Pursuant to the Births and

OF AN ENTRY
Deaths Registration Act 1953

DEATH	Entry No.

Registration district	Administrative area

Sub-district

1. Date and place of death

2. Name and surname	3. Sex
	4. Maiden surname of woman who has married

5. Date and place of birth

6. Occupation and usual address

7. (a) Name and surname of informant	(b) Qualification

(c) Usual address

8. Cause of death

9. I certify that the particulars given by me above are true to the best of my knowledge and belief.

....
Signature
of informant

10. Date of registration	11. Signature of registrar

Certified to be a true copy of an entry in a register in my custody.

....Registrar ....Date **IU   0472**

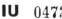

6

G.R.O. 2
STILL-BIRTH Registered in the district of

1	Date of still-birth	:	
2	Place of still-birth	:	
3	Sex	:	
4	Cause of still-birth	:	

5	Father - Name & surname	:	
6	- Occupation	:	
7	Mother - Name & surname	:	
8	- Usual address	:	
9	- Maiden surname	:	
10	- Surname at marriage	:	
	(if different from maiden surname)		
11	Informant - Qualification	:	
12	- Address	:	
	(if different from that at 8 above)		
13	- Signature		
14	Date of registration	:	
15	Signature of Registrar	:	Registrar

District of Registration :	STILL-BIRTH	Ref. No.

CONFIDENTIAL

In all cases:—   Mother's date & place of birth: Age at birth of child

Where parents are
married to each other:—   Father's date & place of birth: Age at birth of child
Date and place of marriage: Duration of marriage
Has the mother been married more than once?
How many children has the mother previously had by her present husband and
by any former husband? (excluding birth or births now being registered):   Live-born
                                                                            Still-born
If multiple birth, give other reference number(s):

HMSO 8091920 11/91 C5 158 67334

7A

Form 6

CERTIFICATE OF STILL-BIRTH

This certificate must be delivered to the Registrar of Births, Deaths and Marriages when the still-birth is registered. It is not an authority for burial or cremation. See the back of this form for notes about registration of a still-birth. Section 56(1) of the Registration of Births, Deaths and Marriages (Scotland) Act 1965, as amended by section 1(2) of the Still-Birth (Definition) Act 1992, defines "still-born child" as meaning "a child which has issued forth from its mother after the twenty fourth week of pregnancy and which did not at any time after being completely expelled from its mother breathe or show any other signs of life", and provides that the expression "still-birth" shall be construed accordingly.

To the Registrar of Births, Deaths and Marriages

*I was present at the still-birth of a *male/female child born
*I have examined the body of a *male/female child which I am informed and believe was still-born

{ *Delete whichever does not apply*

at .... hours, on .... 19 ....
       time   *date*

to ....
       name of mother

at ....
       place of still-birth

I hereby certify that the child was **not born alive** and that, to the best of my knowledge and belief, the cause or probable cause of death, and the estimated duration of pregnancy of the mother were as stated below.

CAUSE OF DEATH *(Please print child)*

I	
Fetal or maternal condition directly causing death	*(a)* .... due to
Antecedent causes	*(b)* .... due to
Fetal or maternal conditions, if any, giving rise to the above cause, the underlying condition to be stated last	*(c)* ....
II	
Other significant conditions of fetus or mother contributing to the death, but not related to the disease or condition causing it	II ....

Registrar to enter

Dist. No. ....

Year. ....

Entry No. ....

Not to be entered in register
Estimated duration of pregnancy

.... *weeks*

Weight of fetus if known

.... *grams*

Signature .... *date* ....

Please ring appropriate letter:-

Certified cause takes account of post-mortem information	A
Information from post-mortem may be available later	B
Post-mortem not proposed	C

A   *Name in* **BLOCK CAPITALS.** ....

B   *Registered medical qualifications or regd. no.* .... *if a registered midwife.*

C   *Address* ....

B2(R)
892

7B   NOTES ABOUT REGISTRATION OF A STILL-BIRTH

A still-birth may be registered either in the **Registration District** where it takes place (the district of occurrence) or in such other registration district in **Scotland** where the mother has her usual residence at the time of the still-birth. Usual residence for this purpose means the address of the parental home and not a temporary address at which the mother may reside for a short period before and after the still-birth e.g. her own mother's home.

Persons required to give information for the registration of a still-born child are:-

   a the father (of a legitimate child only);

   b the mother;

or in the case of the death or inability of the father and mother:-

   c a relative of either parent being a relative who has knowledge of the still-birth;

   d the occupier of the premises in which the child was, to the knowledge of that occupier, still-born;

   e any person present at the still-birth.

8A

MEDICAL CERTIFICATE OF CAUSE OF DEATH   FORM 11

This certificate is intended for the use of the Registrar of Births, Deaths and Marriages, and all persons are warned against accepting or using this certificate for any other purpose. See back of this form for notes about registration of a death.

To the Registrar of Births, Deaths and Marriages

Name of deceased . . . .

Day	Month	Year

Date of death . . . .   Time of death . . . . hours
(Enter approximate time it exact time not known)

Place of death . . . .

I hereby certify that to the best of my knowledge and belief, the cause of death and duration of disease were as stated below.

CAUSE OF DEATH   *(PLEASE PRINT CLEARLY)*

Registrar to enter

District no . . . .

Year . . . .

Entry no . . . .

Not to be entered in register

Approximate interval between onset and death

years	months	days

I

Disease or condition directly leading to death*

a . . . .
  due to (or as a consequence of)

Antecedent causes
Morbid conditions, if any, giving rise to the above cause, the **underlying** condition to be stated **last**

b . . . .
  due to (or as a consequence of)

c . . . .

II

Other significant conditions contributing to the death, but not related to the disease or condition causing it

SPECIMEN

* *This does not mean the mode of dying such as heart failure, asthenia, etc; it means the disease, injury or complication which caused death.*

Please ring the appropriate letter and appropriate figures:—

Certified cause takes account of post-mortem information ...... A
Information from post-mortem may be available later ...... B
Post-mortem not proposed C

Seen after death by me 1
Seen after death by another medical practitioner but not by me 2
Not seen after death by a medical practitioner 3

The deceased woman died during pregnancy
or within six weeks thereafter 1
The deceased woman died between six weeks
and twelve months after pregnancy 2

Please tick box if appropriate
I may be in a position later to give, if asked by the Registrar
General, additional information as to the cause of this death for
the purpose of more precise statistical classification [ ] [ ]

Procurator Fiscal has been informed

Signature ....

Date .... 19 ...

Name in BLOCK
CAPITALS ....

Registered medical qualifications ....

Address ....

For a death in hospital
Name of consultant responsible
for deceased as a patient ....

8B NOTES ABOUT REGISTRATION OF A DEATH

A death may be registered either in the registration district where it takes place (the district of its occurrence) or in such other registration district in Scotland where the deceased person had h s usual residence immediately before his death.

Usual residence for this purpose means the deceased person's permanent home and not an address (e.g. a holiday address) at which he may have been staying temporarily at the time of his death.

Persons required to give information for the registration of a death are:

a   any relative of the deceased;

b   any person present at the death;

c   the deceased's executor or other legal representative;

d   the occupier, at the time of death, of the premises where the death took place;

e   if there is no such person as aforesaid, any other person having knowledge of the particulars to be registered.

N.B.   The word "occupier" includes the governor, keeper, matron, superintendent or other person in charge of a prison, hospital or other institution, and, in relation to a house, includes any person residing therein.

SPECIMEN

APPENDIX 2
— Documentation

9A

Registration of Births, Deaths and Marriages (Scotland) Act 1965

DECLARATION AS TO PARENTAGE BY MOTHER

(To be made before a justice of the peace, notary public or other person authorised by law to administer oaths)

I ....

residing at ....

DO HEREBY SOLEMNLY AND SINCERELY DECLARE that..............................

....

whose usual address is..

is the father of the .... male child named ....

....

and born to me on...19..

at..

AND I make this solemn declaration conscientiously believing the same to be true, and by virtue of the provisions of the Statutory Declarations Act 1835

Dated this............................... day of......................... 19...

Signature ....

Signed and
declared
before me
{
Signature...................................... Date .../.../ 19...

Full Name in Block Letters...

Designation..

Address..
}

(OVER

9B

Section 18 of the Registration of Births, Deaths and Marriages (Scotland) Act 1965 provides that:—

"18.—(1) No person who is not married to the mother of a child and has not been married to her since the child's conception shall be required, as father of the child, to give information concerning the birth of the child and, save as provided in section 20 of this Act, the registrar shall not enter in the register the name and surname of any such person as father of the child except —

(a) at the joint request of the mother and the person acknowledging himself to be the father of the child (in which case that person shall sign the register together with the mother); or

(b) at the request of the mother —

(i) on the production of —

(aa) a declaration in the prescribed form made by the mother stating that that person is the father of the child; and

(bb) a statutory declaration made by that person acknowledging himself to be the father of the child; or

(ii) on production of a decree by a competent court finding or declaring that person to be the father of the child; or

(c) at the request of that person on production of —

(i) a declaration in the prescribed form by that person acknowledging himself to be the father of the child; and

(ii) a statutory declaration made by the mother stating that that person is the father of the child.

(1A) Where a person acknowledging himself to be the father of a child makes a request to the registrar in accordance with paragraph (c) of subsection (1) of this section, he shall be treated as a qualified informant concerning the birth of the child for the purposes of this Act; and the giving of information concerning the birth of the child by that person and the signing of the register by him in the presence of the registrar shall act as a discharge of any duty of any other qualified informant under section 14 of this Act.

(2)   In any case where the name and surname of the father of a child has not been entered in the register, the Registrar General may record that name and surname by causing an appropriate entry to be made in the Register of Corrections Etc. —

(a) if a decree of paternity has been granted by a competent court; or

(b) if there is produced to him a declaration and a statutory declaration such as are mentioned in paragraph (b) or (c) of subsection (1) of this section, and

(c) if, where the mother is dead or cannot be found or is incapable of making a request under subsection (1)(b) of this section, or a declaration under subsection (1)(b)(i)(aa) of this section, or a statutory declaration under subsection (1)(c)(ii) of this section, he is ordered so to do by the sheriff upon application made to the sheriff by the person acknowledging himself to be the father of the child.

Where a decree of paternity has been granted by any court the clerk of court shall, where no appeal has been made against such decree, on the expiration of the time within which such an appeal may be made, or where an appeal has been made against such a decree, on the conclusion of any appellate proceedings, notify the import of such decree in the prescribed form to the Registrar General."

RE 031068 9/86 TBL

10A

Form D

Registration of Births, Deaths and Marriages (Scotland) Act 1965

DECLARATION AS TO PARENTAGE BY FATHER

(To be made before a justice of the peace, notary public or other person authorised by law to administer oaths)

I . . . .

residing at . . . .

DO HEREBY SOLEMNLY AND SINCERELY DECLARE that I am the father of the . . . . . . .male chi

named . . . .

and born on . . . . .19 . .

at . . . .

to . . . .

whose usual address is . . . .

AND I make this solemn declaration conscientiously believing the same to be true, and by virtue of the provisions of the Statutory Declarations Act 1835

Dated this . . . . day of . . . . 19 . .

Signature . . . .

Signature . . . . Date . . ./ . . ./ 19 . .

**Signed and
declared
before me**

Full Name in Block Letters . . . .

Designation . . . .

Address . . . .

(OVE

10B

Section 18 of the Registration of Births, Deaths and Marriages (Scotland) Act 1965 provides that:—

"18.—(1) No person who is not married to the mother of a child and has not been married to her since the child's conception shall be required, as father of the child, to give information concerning the birth of the child and, save as provided in section 20 of this Act, the registrar shall not enter in the register the name and surname of any such person as father of the child except —

(a) at the joint request of the mother and the person acknowledging himself to be the father of the child (in which case that person shall sign the register together with the mother); or

(b) at the request of the mother —

(i) on the production of —

(aa) a declaration in the prescribed form made by the mother stating that that person is the father of the child; and

(bb) a statutory declaration made by that person acknowledging himself to be the father of the child; or

(ii) on production of a decree by a competent court finding or declaring that person to be the father of the child; or

(c) at the request of that person on production of —

(i) a declaration in the prescribed form by that person acknowledging himself to be the father of the child; and

(ii) a statutory declaration made by the mother stating that that person is the father of the child.

(1A) Where a person acknowledging himself to be the father of a child makes a request to the registrar in accordance with paragraph (c) of subsection (1) of this section, he shall be treated as a qualified informant concerning the birth of the child for the purposes of this Act and the giving of information concerning the birth of the child by that person and the signing of the register by him in the presence of the registrar shall act as a discharge of any duty of any other qualified informant under section 14 of this Act.

(2) In any case where the name and surname of the father of a child has not been entered in the register, the Registrar General may record that name and surname by causing an appropriate entry to be made in the Register of Corrections Etc. —

(a) if a decree of paternity has been granted by a competent court; or

(b) if there is produced to him a declaration and a statutory declaration such as are mentioned in paragraph (b) or (c) of subsection (1) of this section, and

(c) if, where the mother is dead or cannot be found or is incapable of making a request under subsection (1)(b) of this section, or a declaration under subsection (1)(b)(i)(aa) of this section, or a statutory declaration under subsection (1)(c)(ii) of this section, he is ordered so to do by the sheriff upon application made to the sheriff by the person acknowledging himself to be the father of the child.

Where a decree of paternity has been granted by any court the clerk of court shall, where no appeal has been made against such decree, on the expiration of the time within which such an appeal may be made, or where an appeal has been made against such a decree, on the conclusion of any appellate proceedings, notify the import of such decree in the prescribed form to the Registrar General."

Ed. Rep. 032528/1 5m 4/87

APPENDIX 2 — Documentation

11A   Form 2

DECLARATION BY THE MOTHER OF A CHILD WHOSE PARENTS ARE NOT MARRIED TO EACH OTHER

(Section 18(1)(b)(i)(aa) and (2)(b) of the Registration of Births, Deaths and Marriages (Scotland Act 1965)

- This declaration must be accompanied by a statutory declaration by the person name above as the father acknowledging himself to be the father of the child.

- The attention of any person making a declaration as aforesaid is drawn to th provisions of section 53(1) of the Registration of Births, Deaths and Marriage (Scotland) Act 1965 (reproduced overleaf).

I ....

residing at ....

DO HEREBY SOLEMNLY AND SINCERELY DECLARE THAT ....

....

whose usual address is ....

is the father of the female/male child name ....

....

born to me on ....

at ....

Dated this .... day of ....

....
Signature

Declared before me at ....

on the ....

day of ....

....Registrar f

the registration district of ....

Perm/RR36/103

11B

THE REGISTRATION OF BIRTHS, DEATHS AND MARRIAGES (SCOTLAND) ACT 1965

"53.-(1)   If any person commits any of the following offences, that is to say -

(a) if he knowingly gives to a district registrar information which is false in a material particular;

(b) if he falsifies or forges any extract, certificate or declaration issued or made, or purporting to be issued or made, under this Act; or

(c) if he knowingly uses, or gives or sends to any person, as genuine any false or forged extract, certificate or declaration issued or made, or purporting to be issued or made, under this Act,

he shall be liable

(i) on conviction on indictment, to a fine or imprisonment for a term not exceeding 2 years or to both;

(ii) on summary conviction, to a fine not exceeding *£2,000 or to imprisonment for a term not exceeding 3 months or to both."

*Subject to review

SPECIMEN

APPENDIX 2
– Documentation

Perm/RR36/103

12A

DECLARATION BY THE FATHER OF A CHILD WHOSE PARENTS ARE NOT MARRIED TO EACH OTHER

(Section 18(1)(c)(i and (2)(b) of the Registration of Births, Deaths and Marriages (Scotland Act 1965)

- This declaration must be accompanied by a statutory declaration by the mother stating that the person making the declaration above is the father of the child.

- The attention of any person making a declaration as aforesaid is drawn to the provisions of section 53(1) of the Registration of Births, Deaths and Marriages (Scotland) Act 1965 (reproduced overleaf).

I ....

residing at ....

DO HEREBY SOLEMNLY AND SINCERELY DECLARE that I am the father of the

female/male child named ....

born on ....

at ....

to ....

whose usual address is ....

Dated this .... day of ....

....
Signature

Declared before me at ....

on the ....

day of ....

....Registrar

the registration district of ....

Perm/RR36/103

12B

THE REGISTRATION OF BIRTHS, DEATHS AND MARRIAGES (SCOTLAND) ACT 1965

"53.-(1)   If any person commits any of the following offences, that is to say -

     (a) if he knowingly gives to a district registrar information which is false in a material particular;

     (b) if he falsifies or forges any extract, certificate or declaration issued or made, or purporting to be issued or made, under this Act; or

     (c) if he knowingly uses, or gives or sends to any person, as genuine any false or forged extract, certificate or declaration issued or made, or purporting to be issued or made, under this Act,

he shall be liable

     (i) on conviction on indictment, to a fine or imprisonment for a term not exceeding 2 years or to both;

     (ii) on summary conviction, to a fine not exceeding *£2,000 or to imprisonment for a term not exceeding 3 months or to both."

*Subject to review

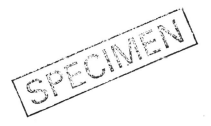

Perm/RR36/103

Index

Entries in **bold** refer to major references. Entries in *italic* refer to figures and tables.